DRCOG Practice Exams: Revision Made Easy

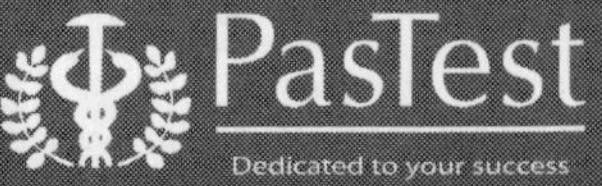

Dedication

To Miss Sikhalo Mabhena for all the love and care, my living stars Sobukhosi and Nqobile.
SN

To my family especially to Anant.
PS

DRCOG Practice Exams: Revision Made Easy

Solwayo Ngwenya MB ChB, DFFP, MRCOG
Senior Registrar in Obstetrics and Gynaecology
Mpilo Central Hospital
Senior Lecturer in Obstetrics and Gynaecology
Faculty of Medicine
National University of Science and Technology
Bulawayo
Zimbabwe

Pinki Singh MB BS, DGO, DNB, MRCOG
Specialist Registrar in Obstetrics and Gynaecology
West Midlands Deanery
United Kingdom

Edited by

Stephen W Lindow MB ChB, MMed(O&G), MD, FCOG(SA), FRCOG
Senior Lecturer in Perinatology
University of Hull
Honorary Consultant Obstetrics and Gynaecology
Hull Royal Infirmary
Hull
United Kingdom

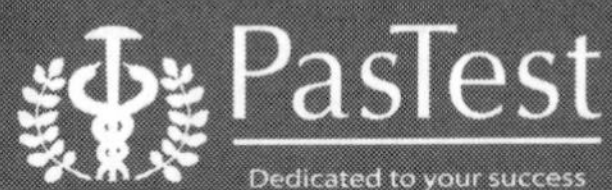

Egerton Court
Parkgate Estate
Knutsford
Cheshire
WA16 8DX

Telephone: 01565 752000

First Published 2007

ISBN: 1 905635 42 7
ISBN: 978 1 905635 42 9
A catalogue record for this book is available from the British Library.

Text prepared by Carnegie Book Production, Lancaster

Printed and bound by Athenaeum Press, Gateshead

Contents

Acknowledgements

The authors would like to thank Michael Dooley, Ali Elfara and Michael Savvas for their contribution to the 2nd edition. We would like to thank Cathy Dickens and Geeta Mehta of PasTest for their invaluable support.

Introduction

This book is designed for candidates preparing to take the Diploma examination of the Royal College of Obstetricians and Gynaecologists (DRCOG).

The Royal College has given permission for the DRCOG syllabus to be reproduced to assist candidates.

From October 2007 the format of the examination has changed and will consist of:

- 18 'best of 5' multiple choice questions to be completed in 30 minutes (12.9% of total marks)
- 40 true/false multiple choice questions to be completed in 90 minutes (57.1% of total marks)
- 30 extended matching questions to be completed in 60 minutes (30% of total marks)

This book has been prepared to reflect the change in the exam format and prepare candidates to demonstrate their knowledge to the full potential.

The questions range from relatively easy to some more demanding and some difficult questions to enable a candidate to test their knowledge thoroughly.

The authors would also stress that there are no short cuts to examination success and preparation is the key.

Good luck.

Stephen Lindow

DRCOG Syllabus

The DRCOG examination is an assessment of knowledge and competence in the subjects of obstetrics, gynaecology, sexual health and family planning at a level appropriate for a general practitioner (GP) in the UK.

Module 1: Basic Clinical Skills

You should understand and know about:

- the patterns of symptoms in women presenting with obstetric or gynaecological problems or sexually transmitted infections and patients in a family planning setting
- the pathophysiological basis of physical signs
- the indications, risks, benefits and effectiveness of investigations in a clinical setting.

You should be aware of relevant ethical and legal issues, including the implications of the legal status of the unborn child, legal issues relating to medical certification and issues related to medical confidentiality. You will be expected to understand the issues surrounding consent in all clinical situations including post-mortem examination and termination of pregnancy.

Module 2: Basic Surgical Skills

You will need to demonstrate an understanding of commonly performed obstetric and gynaecological surgical procedures, including their complications, and the legal issues surrounding consent to surgical procedures.

You should be aware of commonly encountered infections, including an understanding of the principles of infection control.

You will be expected to interpret preoperative investigations and be aware of the principles involved in appropriate preoperative and postoperative care.

Module 3: Antenatal Care

You should understand and demonstrate appropriate knowledge and attitudes in relation to:

- peri-conceptional care, antenatal care and maternal complications of pregnancy
- substance misuse and psychiatric illness
- problems of pregnancy at extremes of reproductive age
- domestic violence in relation to pregnancy.

You should have a good understanding of common medical disorders and the effect that pregnancy may have on them, and also, in turn, their effect on pregnancy. Knowledge of therapeutics in antenatal care is expected.

You should understand the principles of antenatal screening including screening for structural defects, chromosomal abnormalities and haemoglobinopathies and the effects of relevant infections during pregnancy on the fetus and neonate.

Module 4: Management of Labour and Delivery

You should know and understand the initial management of intrapartum problems in a hospital and in a community setting:

- normal and abnormal labour
- interpretation of data and investigations
- induction and augmentation of labour
- assessment of fetal wellbeing and compromise.

An understanding of the management of all obstetric emergencies is expected. You will need to demonstrate appropriate knowledge of regional anaesthesia, analgesia and operative delivery including caesarean section.

Module 5: Postpartum Problems (the Puerperium) Including Neonatal Problems

You should be able to demonstrate appropriate knowledge, management skills and attitudes in relation to postpartum maternal problems, including:

- the normal and abnormal postpartum period
- postpartum haemorrhage
- therapeutics
- perineal care
- psychological disorders
- infant feeding and breast problems.

You should have an understanding of the investigation and management of immediate neonatal problems including neonatal resuscitation.

Module 6: Gynaecological Problems

You will be expected to demonstrate appropriate knowledge, management skills and attitudes in relation to benign gynaecological problems including:

- urogynaecology
- paediatric and adolescent gynaecology
- endocrine problems
- pelvic pain and abnormal vaginal bleeding. This includes early pregnancy loss, including clinical features, investigation and management of disorders leading to early pregnancy loss – miscarriage (including recurrent), ectopic pregnancy and molar pregnancy.

In addition you should know how to assess and manage common sexually transmitted infections including human immunodeficiency virus (HIV)/ acquired immune deficiency syndrome (AIDS) and be familiar with their modes of transmission and clinical features.

You will be also expected to have appropriate knowledge and understanding of:

- clinical features, investigation and management of premalignant and malignant conditions of the female genital tract
- indications and limitations of screening for premalignant and malignant disease
- options available for palliative and terminal care including relief of symptoms and community support
- epidemiology, aetiology, management and prognosis of male and female fertility problems
- investigation and management of the infertile couple in a primary care setting and assisted reproductive techniques and the legal and ethical implications of these procedures.

Module 7: Fertility Control (Contraception and Termination of Pregnancy)

You will be expected to demonstrate appropriate knowledge, management skills and attitudes in relation to:

- fertility control
- termination of pregnancy
- indications, contraindications, complications, mode of action and efficacy of all reversible and irreversible contraceptive methods
- abortion. You should be familiar with the accompanying laws related to abortion, consent, child protection and the Sexual Offences Act(s).

Practice Paper 1 Questions

BEST OF FIVE QUESTIONS

20 Questions: Time allowed 30 minutes. Please give the single most appropriate answer from the list of alternatives.

1.1 A 60-year-old woman presents with history of postmenopausal bleeding. Ultrasound shows an endometrial thickness of 15 mm. Which one of the following is the most appropriate next step in her management?

- A Cervical smear and colposcopic examination
- B Computed tomography (CT) scan
- C Hysterectomy
- D Hysteroscopy + directed biopsy
- E Reassurance

1.2 A 23-year-old heroin addict attends clinic at 12 weeks' gestation. She is keen to know which one of the following is the most likely problem the baby will face if she is continues to use heroin.

- A Intrauterine growth restriction (IUGR)
- B Prematurity
- C Congenital malformation
- D Stillbirth
- E Neonatal admission for withdrawal symptoms

Answers on pages 41–45

1.3 Which one of the following medicines is not associated with fetal anomalies and therefore can be safely used in pregnancy?

A Sulfonamides

B Dalteparin (low-molecular-weight heparin)

C Indometacin

D β-Blockers

E Cocaine

1.4 A woman delivered vaginally 7 days ago in hospital presents with pyrexia of > 38°C, tender lower abdomen, offensive discharge and uterine size corresponding to 18 weeks. Which one of the following options is the most appropriate management plan?

A Antibiotics as an outpatient

B Hospital admission and ultrasound scan for retained products

C Treatment with oxytocics

D Hospital admission for antibiotics

E Options C and D

1.5 You are counselling a 16-year-old primipara about benefits of breast feeding. Which one of the following benefits needs to be told about with reservations?

A Protects mothers against ovarian and premenopausal breast carcinoma

B Reduces risk of postpartum haemorrhage and aids uterine involution

C Highly effective contraceptive

D Protects babies against ear infections and chest infections

E Reduces risk of allergies and juvenile-onset diabetes

1.6 A 36 weeks pregnant multipara with gestational diabetes and hydramnios has spontaneous rupture of membranes. Which one of the following is most appropriate immediate management plan for her?

A Reassure and wait until contractions start

B Ask to go to hospital next day for induction of labour

C Start antibiotics and await onset of labour

D Ask about fetal movements – if normal wait until 37 weeks

E Examine patient vaginally as soon as possibly after rupture of membrane to rule out cord prolapse

1.7 A single homeless mother with a history of bipolar disorder who delivered 2 weeks ago is brought to you with recent-onset abnormal behaviour, not feeding her baby and saying that the baby does not belong to her. Which one of the following is the most likely diagnosis and treatment option in this case?

- A Maternal blues – needs reassurance and counselling
- B Bipolar disorder – to take lithium and continue breast feeding
- C Postnatal depression – fluoxetine
- D Related to illegal drugs – toxicology screen
- E Puerperal psychosis – antipsychotics

1.8 Following an in vitro fertilisation (IVF) pregnancy a 35-year-old woman is found to have a twin gestation on booking scan. Which one of the following complications is most commonly associated with multiple pregnancy that you will discuss with this patient?

- A Risk of congenital malformation
- B Preterm labour before 37 weeks
- C Risk of postpartum bleeding
- D Twin-to-twin transfusion
- E Interlocking of twins

1.9 A 50-year-old nulliparous women presents with abdominal swelling and pain since 2 weeks. She has a history of breast cancer in her family. On ultrasound there is a pelvic mass with ascites. Her CA125 level is 100. Which one of the following is the most likely diagnosis?

- A Serous cystadenocarcinoma
- B Mucinous cystadenoma
- C Fibroma with Meigs syndrome
- D Secondary metastasis from breast
- E Fibroid uterus with degeneration

1.10 A multigravida with history of preterm delivery presents to your general practice. Which one of the following symptoms/signs is unlikely be a feature of the onset of labour in this patient?

- A Uterine contractions every 2–3 minutes
- B Show
- C Dilatation of cervix > 3 cm
- D Constant backache
- E Tense bag of membranes on vaginal examination

1.11 A 17-year-old girl with body mass index (BMI) of 21 and history of epilepsy complaints of hirsutism. Her periods are regular. Which one of the following is the most likely cause for her hirsutism?

A Cushing syndrome

B Phenytoin

C Granulosa cell tumour

D Polycystic ovarian syndrome (PCOS)

E Congenital adrenal hyperplasia

1.12 A 30-year-old sexually active women with history of insertion of an intrauterine contraceptive device (IUCD) complains of vaginal discharge with a fishy odour. The vaginal pH is > 4.5. Microscopic examination reveals clue cells. Which one of the following is the most appropriate diagnosis?

A Gonorrhoeal infection

B Candidal infection

C Bacterial vaginosis

D Trichomonal infection

E Staphylococcal infection

1.13 An iv drug user presents with vaginal discharge and a painless lesion on the labia. Which one of the following infections is the most likely cause for her symptoms?

A Candidal infection

B Herpes simplex infection

C Trichomonal infection

D Syphilitic ulcer

E Lymphogranuloma venereum

1.14 Which one of the following findings should be taken seriously and further investigated in a pregnant woman?

A Maternal thyroid gland enlargement with minimal changes in free T3 and T4 levels

B Up to 50% increase in plasma volume by 32 weeks of pregnancy

C A rise in blood pressure of 20–30 mmHg of non-pregnant level in second trimester

D Increase in the renal blood flow by 30–50% in the first trimester of pregnancy

E Reduced gastric mobility and gastric secretions

1.15 A 20-year-old woman presents with history of 6 weeks' amenorrhoea, pain and bleeding per vagina. An ultrasound shows no intrauterine gestational sac. Her β human chorionic gonadotrophin (hCG) level is 550 I. u/l which further increases to 700 after 48 hours. Which one of the following is the most appropriate diagnosis in this case.

- A Missed miscarriage
- B Early normal pregnancy
- C Ectopic pregnancy
- D Complete miscarriage
- E Threatened miscarriage

1.16 In an antenatal patient, which one of the following issues should not be a worry to you and could be managed by just reassuring the patient?

- A Blood pressure > 140/90 mmHg
- B Haemorrhage after 24 weeks of pregnancy
- C Transverse lie at 32 weeks
- D Calf pain and swelling
- E Reduced fetal movements

1.17 A couple has been trying for a baby for 3 years. The female partner has history of dysmenorrhoea and heavy and painful periods. Which one of the following should not be a part of management for this couple?

A Investigation for infertility, which can be justified based on inability to conceive after 1 year of unprotected intercourse

B Semen analysis as initial investigation for couple seeking treatment

C Serum progesterone levels to check ovulation

D Laparoscopy and dye test

E Drug treatment for endometriosis-related infertility

1.18 A 29-year-old woman with a BMI of 35 and oligomenorrhoea is trying for a baby. Which one of the following is the most appropriate management plan for her?

A Clomifene

B In vitro fertilisation

C Weight loss

D Gonadotrophin treatment is first line treatment for patient with anovulation

E Management should be directed at correcting biochemical (hormonal) abnormalities

1.19 A 65-year-old menopausal woman with history of myocardial infarction and diabetes presents with complaints related to prolapse. On examination you find a cystocele. Which one of the following treatment options would you like to offer her?

A Vaginal hysterectomy

B Ring pessary

C Round ligament placation, as it provides important support to uterus

D Oestrogen-based hormone replacement therapy, which is proven to help prevent prolapse in menopausal women

E Fothergill repair, which is best suited for women who have completed their family

1.20 A 31-year-old anxious women is 6 weeks pregnant and enquires about prenatal diagnostic tests. While counselling her which one of the following would be the most appropriate statement?

A Amniocentesis is usually done between 13 and 15 weeks' gestation

B Full karyotype results of amniocentesis specimens take approximately 3 weeks

C Amniocentesis should be offered to her as she is more than 30 years old

D Procedure-related risk of fetal loss following chorion villus sampling is 4%

E Limb defects may occur if chorion villus sampling is carried out after 11 weeks' gestation

MULTIPLE CHOICE QUESTIONS

40 Questions: Time allowed 1½ hours. Indicate your answers clearly by putting a tick against the correct or true options and a cross against the incorrect or false options. (The section on answers in this book lists the correct (true) options.)

1.21 Which of the following statements about fetal cardiotocography is/are true?

- A Fetal heart rate decreases with increasing gestational age
- B The normal baseline heart rate in late pregnancy is between 120 and 150 bpm
- C Baseline tachycardia can be associated with maternal fever
- D Heart rate variability increases with increasing gestational age
- E Late decelerations and reduced variability are associated with fetal hypoxia

1.22 Dyspareunia:

- A Is classified as superficial when pain occurs after penetration
- B Can be caused by a urethral caruncle
- C Is associated with vaginal lactobacilli
- D Is associated with atrophic vaginitis
- E May require a laparoscopy to aid the diagnosis

Answers on pages 47–65

1.23 Anti-D prophylaxis should be given to all non-sensitised rhesus-D-negative women after the following events in the third trimester:

- A Eclamptic fit
- B HELLP (haemolysis, elevated liver enzymes and a low platelet count) syndrome
- C Transvaginal scan
- D Premature labour
- E Abdominal trauma

1.24 Endometrial biopsy:

- A Should be restricted to women over the age of 35 years
- B Should be carried out before the commencement of hormone replacement therapy
- C Always requires an anaesthetic
- D Is mandatory in women on unopposed oestrogen who have an intact uterus
- E Is mainly used to detect endometrial polyps

1.25 Diagnostic tests for Down syndrome include:

- A Chorionic villus sampling
- B α-fetoprotein testing
- C A combination of α-fetoprotein, β-human chorionic gonadotrophin and oestriol testing in maternal serum
- D Amniocentesis
- E Ultrasound scanning at 12 weeks' gestation

1.26 Which of the following statements about pelvic inflammatory disease (PID) is/are true?

- A It is considered a sexually transmitted disease
- B The incidence is about 1 per 1000 in all women between the ages of 15 and 39
- C About 15% of all women will have had PID by the age of 30
- D It is now widely accepted as polymicrobial in origin
- E Chronic PID is a rare complaint

1.27 Breech presentation may be due to:

- A Bicornuate uterus
- B Hydrocephalus
- C Polyhydramnios
- D Placenta praevia
- E Prematurity

1.28 The progestogen-only pill method of contraception is particularly indicated in:

- A Women over 35 who smoke
- B Women with endometriosis
- C During lactation
- D Women with hyperemesis
- E Women with diabetes

1.29 Which of the following recommendations for the management of a woman with suspected varicella contact in pregnancy is/are true?

A If a pregnant woman has had a significant contact with but has no history of varicella infection check the varicella immunoglobulin G (IgG) in the serum

B If a pregnant woman is not immune to varicella zoster and an infection occurs before 20 weeks' gestation she should be given varicella zoster IgG as soon as possible

C Detection of IgG in maternal serum indicates primary varicella zoster infection

D If a woman develops primary varicella in the first 20 weeks of pregnancy then there is a 2% risk of congenital varicella infection

E If there is no history of varicella and the contact occurs after 20 weeks there is no risk of congenital varicella infection

1.30 Amenorrhoea can be caused by:

A Hypogonadotrophic hypogonadism

B Anaemia

C Hypoprolactinaemia

D Turner syndrome

E Asherman syndrome

1.31 Women of African origin have an increased risk for:

A Fibroids

B Endometriosis

C Ectopic pregnancy

D Severe pre-eclampsia

E Postmenopausal osteoporosis

1.32 The following can induce ovulation:

A Clomifene citrate

B Ethinylestradiol

C Medroxyprogesterone acetate

D Human chorionic gonadotrophin

E Human menopausal gonadotrophin

1.33 Anti-D should be given:

A To all women with threatened abortion

B To a rhesus-negative woman who has just delivered

C To a rhesus-negative woman 2 weeks' post partum

D During an in vitro fertilisation cycle

E At the time of amniocentesis in rhesus-negative women

1.34 The use of progestogen-only contraceptives is governed by the following considerations:

A Ovulation is not always inhibited

B Protection against pregnancy is as good as with the combined pill

C There is a substantial risk in older women of thromboembolic phenomena

D Uterine bleeding may become irregular

E The dose of progestogen is much larger than in the combined pill

1.35 Magnesium sulphate:

A Is used in the management of intrauterine growth retardation

B Is used in the prevention of eclampsia

C Can cause loss of deep tendon reflexes

D Can cause loss of respiratory depression

E Has a therapeutic range between 30 mmol/l and 40 mmol/l

1.36 A pulmonary embolism should be suspected if there is:

A A painful calf

B Haemoptysis

C Pyrexia

D Hypertension

E A dry cough

1.37 Which of following statements regarding advice on preventing deep vein thrombosis for pregnant women travelling by air is/are correct?

A There is good, direct, evidence-based data to guide thromboprophylactic advice for pregnant air travellers

B An increase in body mass index is not an additional risk factor

C Women with a past history or strong family history of deep vein thrombosis should consume minimal alcohol and coffee during air travel

D Women with multiple pregnancies should consider low-molecular-weight heparin on a long-haul flight, on the day of travel and the day after

E Low-dose aspirin 75 mg/day for 3 days before travel and on the day of travel is an acceptable alternative in those who cannot take low-molecular-weight heparin

1.38 Which of the following statements about the cause of subfertility is/are true?

A Endometriosis is found in about 25% of cases

B Ovulatory failure accounts for about 20% of cases

C Sperm defects are found in about 5% of couples

D Tubal damage is the most common cause in females

E A cause is found after standard investigations in about 70% of cases

1.39 Recognised causes of neonatal fits include:

A Hypoglycaemia

B Birth trauma

C Meningitis

D Down syndrome

E Bottle feeding

1.40 Which of the following statements about semen analysis is/are true?

A Normal volume is between 2 ml and 5 ml

B Aspermia may be due to retrograde ejaculation

C Asthenospermia means decreased motility

D Motility is usually greater than 40%

E Analysis should be done 10–12 days after the last ejaculation

1.41 Causes of anovulation include:

A Hypoprolactinaemia

B Polycystic ovarian syndrome

C Premature menopause

D Hypothalamic hypogonadism

E Wedge resection of the ovaries

1.42 With regard to endometriosis:

A It is defined as functional endometrial tissue lying outside the uterine cavity

B Histological examination of deposits for glands and stroma is essential to reach a clinical dignosis of endometriosis

C It is always symptomatic

D It has an incidence of about 10%, which is increasing

E It is always associated with subfertility

1.43 Primary cytomegalovirus infection in pregnancy may cause which of the following in the fetus?

A Microcephaly

B Blood dyscrasias

C Myocarditis

D Pneumonia

E Enterocolitis

1.44 With regard to reversal of sterilisation:

A It is requested by about 10% of women

B It has an ectopic rate of about 3%

C If a Filshie clip has been applied, it is successful in approximately 70% of cases

D The rate of success rises when an operating microscope is used

E It should only be considered if the patient's serum follicle-stimulating hormone level is > 20 IU/l.

1.45 Relative contraindications for a laparoscopy include:

A A positive pregnancy test

B Previous pulmonary embolism

C Chronic tuberculous peritonitis

D A diaphragmatic hernia

E Previous hysterectomy

1.46 Which of the following statements is/are true regarding the healthy neonate?

A The onset of physiological jaundice is between the sixth and eighth day

B The bowel is sterile at birth

C Urine is not normally passed until 24 hours after birth

D The respiratory rate is in the region of 25–35/min

E The ductus arteriosus closes functionally within an hour of birth

1.47 Endometrial carcinoma:

A Is more common in obese women

B Is a squamous carcinoma in most cases

C Is more common in diabetic women

D Can be excluded if a cervical smear is normal

E Is more common in postmenopausal women receiving cyclical oestrogen and progestogen hormone replacement therapy

1.48 Cephalopelvic disproportion:

- A Exists when the capacity of the birth canal is insufficient for safe vaginal delivery of the fetus with a cephalic presentation
- B Can usually be diagnosed antenatally by abdominal palpation
- C May be associated with non-engagement of the head at term
- D Is accurately diagnosed by X-ray pelvimetry
- E Often occurs with a brow presentation

1.49 Polyhydramnios may be due to:

- A Potter syndrome
- B Oesophageal atresia
- C An open neural tube defect
- D Turner syndrome
- E Ovarian hyperstimulation syndrome

1.50 Preterm birth:

- A Is defined as delivery of an infant between 24 and 37 completed weeks
- B Occurs in about 1% of all births
- C Is due to multiple pregnancy in 6% of cases
- D Is associated with congenital uterine abnormalities
- E Can be prevented in 70% of occasions by tocolytics

1.51 Which of the following complications of pregnancy is/are associated with bacterial vaginosis?

A Gestational diabetes

B Pre-eclampsia

C Prolonged pregnancy

D Low birth weight

E Preterm labour

1.52 At antenatal booking, women should:

A Have been informed of the hospital's antenatal plan and advised to follow it

B Be advised not to wear a seat belt

C Have their body mass index measured

D Have a psychiatric history taken

E Be encouraged to have HIV screening

1.53 What advice should be given to pregnant women?

A Sexual activity should be reduced

B Maternal smoking should be reduced because it reduces average birth weight

C Excessive alcohol consumption by the mother can be associated with fetal growth retardation

D Women with previous growth-retarded infants should not continue to work during any future pregnancy

E Folic acid should be taken in a dose of 4 mg/day by all pregnant women

1.54 Which of the following statements about pelvic inflammatory disease (PID) is/are true?

A PID is often due to *Mycoplasma hominis*

B About 20% of women who have it are infertile

C About 20% of women who have it develop chronic pelvic pain

D The prevalence is greater among women from higher socioeconomic strata

E Prevalence is increased in African/African Caribbean women

1.55 Iron supplements given in pregnancy to prevent anaemia:

A Reduce the incidence of proteinuric hypertension

B Reduce the incidence of antepartum haemorrhage

C Reduce the incidence of maternal infection

D Decrease the incidence of preterm delivery

E Decrease the incidence of intrauterine growth retardation

1.56 With regard to ovarian hyperstimulation syndrome (OHSS):

A It is an iatrogenic condition

B If no pregnancy occurs, the syndrome will typically resolve in 2 months time

C The treatment of OHSS is often careful observation

D Severe OHSS is characterised by the presence of free intraperitoneal fluid, pleural effusions and oliguria

E The prevalence of mild and moderate forms of OHSS is < 1% in all women undergoing ovulation induction

1.57 With regard to postnatal mental illnesses:

A Postnatal blues occur in 50–80% of all women who give birth

B Postnatal psychosis affects 10–20% of women in the postpartum period

C Postnatal depression occurs in 0.2% of all women who give birth

D The rate of recurrence postnatal psychosis in the next pregnancy is 20%

E The blues are characterised by a considerable mood swings and disturbances in perception

1.58 With regard to electronic fetal monitoring:

A Normal fetal heart baseline rate is between 120 and 150 beats per minute

B The cardiotocography recording speeds vary from 2 cm/min to 5 cm/min

C Ritodrine is associated with a reduced fetal heart rate

D Magnesium sulphate causes a decrease in fetal heart rate variability

E The prevalence of cerebral palsy from intrapartum events is about 1%

1.59 Which of the following statements is/are true?

- A By 2025 the number of people aged over 65 will have risen from 420 million in 2000 to 825 million
- B The definition of the menopause is 'the permanent cessation of menstruation resulting from the loss of pituitary activity'
- C The climacteric is the phase which marks the transition from the reproductive to the non-reproductive state
- D Premature menopause is said to occur if menses ceases before the age of 47
- E The menopause is caused by ovarian failure

1.60 A 38-year-old woman presents with menorrhagia and dysmenorrhoea 4 years after being sterilised by the Filshie clip method. She needs three boxes of tampons for each period. No abnormality is found on pelvic examination. With regard to this case:

- A The amount of sanitary protection correlates well with menstrual blood loss
- B The woman's subjective assessment of her blood loss is likely to be reasonably accurate
- C Her menstrual problems are caused by the sterilisation procedure
- D The only effective treatment is a hysterectomy and bilateral salpingo-oophorectomy
- E Anovulation is a likely cause

EXTENDED MATCHING QUESTIONS

30 Questions: Time allowed 1 hour.

THEME: MINOR DISORDERS OF PREGNANCY

A Adrenergic agents
B Antihistamines
C Antacids
D Aspirin
E Explanation and reassurance
F Increased dietary fibre
G Lubricant laxatives
H Paracetamol
I Proton pump inhibitors
H Support stockings

Instructions: From the list above, choose the most appropriate initial management for each minor disorder of pregnancy given below. Each option can be used once, more than once or not at all.

1.61 A woman in the mid-trimester of pregnancy with severe symptoms of heartburn. 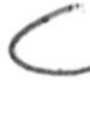

1.62 A 28-week pregnant woman with symphysis pubis dysfunction. 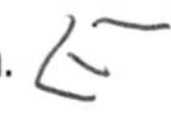

1.63 A woman with constipation and haemorrhoids.

Answers on pages 67–71

THEME: GENITAL TRACT INFECTIONS

A *Chlamydia trachomatis*
B Group B streptococcus
C *Haemophilus ducreyi*
D *Haemophilus influenzae*
E *Staphylococcus aureus*
F *Treponema pallidum*
G *Trichomonas vaginalis*

Instructions: From the list above, choose the organism most likely to be causative of the clinical scenarios given below. Each option can be used once, more than once or not at all.

1.64 A 26-year-old woman presents with a fishy, frothy yellowish vaginal discharge.

1.65 A 19-year-old woman is found at laparoscopy to have severe bilateral tubal damage.

1.66 A sexually active 34-year-old woman develops a soft chancre on her vulva.

THEME: DEEP VENOUS THROMBOSIS IN PREGNANCY

A D-dimer estimation
B Duplex ultrasound
C Low-molecular-weight heparin – subcutaneous
D Unfractionated heparin – subcutaneous
E Unfractionated heparin – intravenous
F Warfarin
G X-ray venogram

Instructions: From the list above, choose the most appropriate management option for the circumstances described below. Each option can be used once, more than once or not at all.

1.67 Initial management of a woman with symptoms and signs suggestive of a deep venous thrombosis in the leg. C

1.68 A woman who needs maintenance therapy for deep vein thrombosis in pregnancy. C

1.69 A woman who needs treatment for an existing deep vein thrombosis. It is 12 hours after a caesarean section and she is thought to be at a high risk for post partum haemorrhage. E

THEME: PRESCRIBING FOR BREAST-FEEDING WOMEN

A Another medication (not mentioned in this list) should be given
B Breast feeding should be discontinued to allow medication to be given.
C Co-amoxiclav and continue breast feeding
D Drug treatment should be withheld
E Erythromycin and continue breast feeding
F Fluoxetine and continue breast feeding
G Oral prednisolone and continue breast feeding
H Warfarin and continue breast feeding

Instructions: From the list above choose the most appropriate management option for a woman who would like to continue breast feeding. Each option can be used once, more than once or not at all.

1.70 A woman with severe postnatal depression.

1.71 A woman with endometritis after a caesarean section.

1.72 Maintenance treatment for deep vein thrombosis.

THEME: SUBFERTILITY

A Hormone profiles
B Cervical smear test
C Laparoscopy and dye test
D Oestrogen levels
E Pelvic ultrasound scan
F Semen analysis
G Sickling test

Instructions: From the list above choose the appropriate investigation for patients presenting with subfertility for each of the situations described below. Each option can be used once, more than once or not at all.

1.73 A 23-year-old woman presents with history of severe pelvic inflammatory disease in the past and primary infertility. C

1.74 A couple presents at their general practice complaining of subfertility. The woman has two children from a previous partner, the current partner has no children and he is 36 years of age. F

1.75 An obese 26-year-old woman with hirsutism presenting with primary subfertility. A

THEME: PRETERM LABOUR

A Allow labour to progress with no suppression of contractions
B Atosiban (oxytocin receptor antagonist) infusion
C Augment labour with oxytocin
D Caesarean section
E Magnesium sulphate infusion
F Nifedipine orally
G Ritodrine infusion

Instructions: From the list above choose the most appropriate management option for the clinical scenarios described below. Each option can be used once, more than once or not at all.

1.76 Symptoms and signs of preterm labour at 26 weeks' gestation. Membranes are intact.

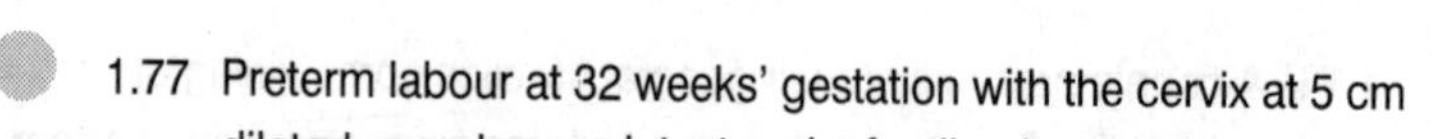

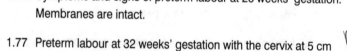

1.77 Preterm labour at 32 weeks' gestation with the cervix at 5 cm dilated, membranes intact and a footling breech presentation.

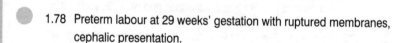

1.78 Preterm labour at 29 weeks' gestation with ruptured membranes, cephalic presentation.

THEME: UTEROVAGINAL PROLAPSE

A Bartholin cyst
B Cystocele
C Enterocele
D Rectocele
E Urethrocele
F Uterine prolapse
G Vaginal cyst
H Vault prolapse

Instructions: Weakness in vaginal and uterine supports can present in different forms. From the list above choose the most likely diagnosis from the list that matches the clinical pictures given below. Each option can be used once, more than once or not at all.

1.79 On examining the vagina of a multiparous woman with a Sims speculum in the left lateral position, a bulge in the upper two-third of the anterior vaginal wall is seen, which increases with coughing.

1.80 A 46-year-old patient presents with feeling a lump in the lower part of posterior vaginal wall and incomplete bowel evacuation. She had a hysterectomy for menorrhagia 4 years ago.

1.81 A 48-year-old woman who still has an intact uterus presents with a history of vague vaginal discomfort and is found to have a swelling in the vagina which produces a gurgling sound on pressure.

THEME: URINARY INCONTINENCE

A Detrusor overactivity
B Ectopic ureter
C Fistula
D Mixed incontinence
E Overflow incontinence
F Urethral caruncle
G Urodynamic stress incontinence

Instructions: Urinary incontinence could have different pathologies. What is the most likely reason for incontinence in the following clinical scenarios? Choose the single mostly likely diagnosis from the list above. Each option can be used once, more than once or not at all.

1.82 A 44-year-old patient presents with urgency and urodynamic studies reveal detrusor contractions during the filling phase when the patient is attempting to inhibit micturition.

1.83 A 25-year-old patient complaining of continuously leaking urine following a forceps delivery for prolonged second stage, 3 weeks previously.

1.84 A demonstrable leak is seen during urodynamic studies when the patient is asked to cough.

THEME: PERINATAL STATISTICS

A < 10%
B 20–30%
C 30–40%
D 50–60%
E 70–80%
F > 90%

Instructions: From the list above give the most accurate estimation related to the current state of medical practice. Each option can be used once, more than once or not at all.

1.85 Incidence of preterm delivery.

1.86 The chance of fetal survival until discharge of a baby born at 26 weeks' gestation who was alive at the onset of labour.

1.87 The chance of fetal survival until discharge of a baby born at 32 weeks' gestation who was alive at the onset of labour.

THEME: ABDOMINAL PAIN

A Acute gastroenteritis
B Fibroid degeneration
C Haematocolpos
D Ovarian hyperstimulation syndrome
E Ovarian torsion
F Pelvic abscess
G Primary dysmenorrhoea
H Secondary dysmenorrhoea
I Ruptured ovarian cyst

Instructions: From the list above choose the most likely cause for acute abdomen in the patients presenting with complains below. Each option can be used once, more than once or not at all.

1.88 A 34-year-old African Caribbean woman with a history of heavy periods complains of acute lower abdominal pain associated with vomiting. B

1.89 A 15-year-old schoolgirl complains of lower abdominal pains preceding menstrual flow that persist for a couple of days. G

1.90 A woman who has had fertility treatment with gonadotrophins presents with vomiting, acute lower abdominal pains and abdominal swelling.

D

Practice Paper 1
Answers

BEST OF FIVE ANSWERS

1.1 D: Hysteroscopy and directed biopsy

Approximately 10% of postmenopausal bleeding cases are due to endometrial cancer. Hysteroscopy + directed biopsy is the standard investigation for diagnosis if the endometrium is thickened. Pipelle sampling can be done in the outpatient clinic if endometrial thickness is more than 5 mm but less than 10 mm.

1.2 E: Neonatal admission for withdrawal symptoms

Use of opiates (heroin, methadone, etc.) in pregnancy is known to be associated with withdrawal symptoms in babies. It is also associated with prematurity, IUGR and stillbirth. However, there is no increased risk of congenital malformations.

1.3 B: Dalteparin (low-molecular-weight heparin)

Low-molecular-weight heparins and heparin do not cross placenta, and therefore are safe for the baby. Warfarin can cause skeletal abnormalities, sulfonamides can cause hyperbilirubinaemia, indometacin can cause premature closure of the ductus arteriosus, β-blockers can cause growth restriction and cocaine can cause placental abruption.

Questions on pages 3–12

1.4 D: Hospital admission for antibiotics

Puerperal pyrexia is defined as rise in temp > 38°C on two or more occasions within 14 days of delivery. The most common cause is endometritis, and others are urinary tract infection (*Escherichia coli*, *Proteus* and *Klebsiella*) breast infections, wound infection from lower segment caesarean section and perineal tears, infected pelvic haematomas and venous thrombosis. Endometritis can also present as a sub-involuted uterus besides the above mentioned presentation. The patient needs to be given iv antibiotics to start with and may need to be investigated, therefore requiring hospital admission.

1.5 C: Highly effective contraceptive

Breast feeding is an effective method of contraception only if the baby is exclusively breast fed. It protects babies against allergies and infections including gastroenteritis, urinary tract infection, and chest and ear infections.

1.6 E: Examine patient vaginally as soon as possibly after rupture of membrane to rule out cord prolapse

Cord prolapse occurs after rupture of membranes and is more likely to occur in multipara with hydramnios. It is more likely in premature preterm rupture of membranes, small preterm fetus polyhydramnios, high head, long cord and malpresentations. Attempts should be made to reach an early diagnosis, to keep the cord in the vagina and to lift the presenting part to avoid compression.

1.7 E: Puerperal psychosis – antipsychotics

Puerperal psychosis is more common in woman after first delivery who have previous bipolar disorder. Onset is typically 2–3 weeks after delivery. Two-thirds of women have baby blues, which occur early in puerperium and are usually self-limiting. Postnatal depression often starts late and has approximately 50–60% risk of recurrence in the next postpartum period.

1.8 B: Preterm labour before 37 weeks

Preterm labour occurs in approximately 40% of twins compared with 5% of singletons. Twin pregnancies have a twice as high rate of congenital malformation as singleton pregnancies. The incidence of twin pregnancy is 11/1000 in UK. All twins should be delivered in units with appropriate facilities and on-site medical help because of the high rate of intrapartum complications.

1.9 A: Serous cystadenocarcinoma

Serous cystadenocarcinoma accounts for 40% of all ovarian malignancies. Mucinous cystadenoma is the commonest benign neoplasm. Ovarian cancer is the second most common cancer in women in the UK. About 1% occur in women with family history of two or more affected first-degree relatives with breast or ovarian malignancy. The risk of ovarian malignancy is reduced by the use of contraceptive pills. The risk is higher in nulliparous women.

1.10 D: Constant backache

All except continuous backache are signs of true labour. Continuous lower abdominal pain or backache is often because of a urinary tract infection or musculoskeletal problems. However, labour and placental abruption should be ruled out in pregnant women presenting with abdominal pain.

1.11 B: Phenytoin

The most likely cause in this case is phenytoin. PCOS causes oligomenorrhoea and is associated with a high BMI. Granulosa cell tumour is an oestrogen-secreting tumour. Hilus cell tumour and gonadoblastoma are androgenic tumours which can cause hirsutism.

1.12 C: Bacterial vaginosis

Vaginal pH > 4.5, clue cells and fishy odour are diagnostic features of bacterial vaginosis. It is more common in sexually active women and IUCD users.

1.13 D: Syphilitic ulcer

Syphilitic ulcers (chancres) are painless. All the other infections can cause vulvitis and pain.

1.14 C: A rise in blood pressure of 20–30 mmHg of non-pregnant level in second trimester

Blood pressure (BP), especially diastolic BP falls by 10–20 mmHg in the mid-trimester, and a rise in BP is not a normal finding. There is an increase in plasma volume, red blood cell mass, glomerular filtration rate and renal blood flow. Free thyroid levels do not change much because of the increased secretion of thyroid-binding globulin.

1.15 C: Ectopic pregnancy

The most likely reason for suboptimal rise in β-hCG is ectopic pregnancy. It usually rises by more than 66% in normal pregnancy. In missed miscarriage and complete miscarriage the levels fall.

1.16 C: Transverse lie at 32 weeks

A transverse lie at 32 weeks is not an indication for referral. It needs referral only after 36 weeks. All other given conditions need referral to hospital.

1.17 E: Drug treatment for endometriosis-related infertility

Surgical treatment has been shown to improve the rate of conception in patients with endometriosis. Investigations for infertility can be started after 1 year. Serum progesterone can only tell in retrospect if ovulation had occurred. Laparoscopy and dye test with possible treatment for endometriosis will aid diagnosis and treatment of endometriosis.

1.18 C: Weight loss

This patient is most likely to have PCOS. The prevalence of PCOS in asymptomatic patients is approximately 25%. Loss of weight in women with high BMI by even 10% can induce regular ovulation. Clomifene is the first line medical treatment for anovulation. Management of PCOS is directed to symptoms rather than biochemical parameters.

1.19 B: Ring pessary

Ring pessary is the safest and best option for a woman with multiple medical co-morbidities. Twenty per cent of all gynaecological operations are for prolapse. Vaginal hysterectomy will not help women with cystocele. Fothergill repair is best for young women with prolapse who want to conserve their uterus. Round ligament placation is not a treatment option for prolapse, and hormone replacement therapy is not beneficial in treatment of prolapse.

1.20 B: Full karyotype results of amniocentesis specimens take approximately 3 weeks

All other statements are incorrect. Amniocentesis is usually performed at 15–16 weeks and has been offered in the past to women > 35 years of age. The rate of procedure-related fetal loss due to amniocentesis is 0.5%, and with chorion villus sampling it is 1–2%. Limb defects occur if chorion villus sampling is done < 10 weeks' of gestation.

MULTIPLE CHOICE ANSWERS

1.21 AC

Is it important to understand cardiotocograms. Baseline tachycardias can be associated with drugs, prematurity, hypoxia or maternal pyrexia. Baseline bradycardia (90–120 bpm) is important if there are also decelerations or decreased variability. Rarely it can be due to congenital heart problems. Severe bradycardia (< 90 bpm) is usually associated with a severely compromised fetus. Chronic hypoxia causes a loss of baseline variability. Early deceleration begins with the onset of a contraction and quickly returns to the baseline before the end of the contraction. It is usually associated with compression of the fetal head and is not an indication of fetal distress. On the other hand, late deceleration is associated with fetal hypoxia and is present when the low point of the deceleration occurs after the peak of the contraction with a slow rate of recovery of the fetal heart. Variable decelerations are sometimes difficult to interpret and can be associated with cord compression.

1.22 BDE

Dyspareunia is pain or difficulty having intercourse. Superficial dyspareunia is defined as pain at the onset of penetration whereas deep dyspareunia is pain that occurs after penetration. Superficial dyspareunia can be associated with vulval, vaginal and urethral disease. Vaginal *Lactobacillus* is part of the normal vaginal flora. Postmenopausal atrophic vaginitis responds well to local oestrogen treatment. Deep dyspareunia is often associated with pelvic pathology, such as pelvic inflammatory disease, endometriosis, ovarian cysts, uterine fibroids and ectopic pregnancy.

Questions on pages 13–27

1.23 E

The following are potentially sensitising events during pregnancy:

- invasive prenatal diagnosis, eg chorionic villus sampling, amniocentesis, fetal blood sampling
- antepartum haemorrhage
- external cephalic version of fetus
- abdominal trauma
- intrauterine death.

1.24 AD

The main purpose of endometrial biopsy is the early detection of endometrial hyperplasia or malignancy. It does not reduce menstrual flow. Biopsies should be restricted to women over the age of 35 as endometrial carcinoma is uncommon in younger women. Before starting hormone replacement therapy there is no need to assess the endometrium routinely unless, of course, there is unexplained abnormal vaginal bleeding. Nowadays with different outpatient procedures including Pipelle and vabra samplings there is usually no need to perform a general anaesthetic. Women with a uterus should not receive unopposed oestrogens because there is an increased risk of endometrial carcinoma and are in need of investigation. Flexible outpatient hysteroscopy with or without endometrial sampling and/or scanning is now an acceptable method of assessing the endometrial cavity.

1.25 AD

Note the term 'diagnostic'. Biochemistry and ultrasound are useful as screening tests.

1.26 AD

PID is considered to be a sexually transmitted infection because sexual intercourse instigates the necessary damage and as the endometrium is always affected it is thought that the infection ascends. The incidence is around 10 per 1000 in all women between the ages of 15 and 39, but may increase to 20 per 1000 in the 15–24-year age group. PID is widely accepted as being polymicrobial in origin. *Chlamydia trachomatis* and *Neisseria gonorrhoea* are the organisms usually transmitted, but others, such as *Mycoplasma hominis*, *Mycoplasma genitalis* and *Ureaplasma urealyticum*, may be implicated. The organisms of the endogenous flora of the lower genital tract often act as secondary pathogens. These include group B streptococci, *Escherichia coli*, *Gardnerella vaginalis*, *Clostridium* spp., *Actinomyces* and *Bacteroides* spp. Chronic PID is a very common complaint with those having had an episode carrying a six to ten times risk of further episodes. There is a 1:6 chance of tubal infertility, a seven-fold increase of ectopic pregnancy, a 1:5 chance of deep dyspareunia and a 4:5 chance of menstrual disturbances.

1.27 ABCDE

There are many causes of breech presentation:

- Maternal causes:
  - Grand multiparity
  - Uterine abnormalities, including bicornuate uterus
  - Pelvic tumours, including ovarian cysts and fibroids
  - Severe bony pelvic abnormality
- Fetal problems:
  - Prematurity – the prevalence of breech presentation decreases from about 15% at 29–32 weeks' gestation to 3–4% at delivery
  - Multiple pregnancy
  - Fetal abnormality which could be associated with polyhydramnios, oligohydramnios or hydrocephalus
- Placenta praevia

1.28 ACDE

Current evidence suggests progestogen-only pill can be continued in smokers. Progestogen-only pill should not be chosen in preference to the combined contraceptive pill in women with endometriosis as it does not reliably suppress endogenous oestrogen. Diabetic women tolerate the progestogen-only pill, resulting in good compliance. In obese women efficacy is a concern. As a working rule, Professor John Guillebaud in his book *Contraception – Your Questions Answered* states: 'Contraindications to or side-effects with the combined oral contraceptive pill, and a hormonal method is preferred? Try the progestogen-only pill.'

1.29 ABDE

At least 85% of women will have had varicella and will be positive for IgG. Detection of IgM in maternal serum indicates primary varicella infection. Referral to a specialist centre for detailed ultrasound examination at 16–20 weeks' gestation or 5 weeks after infection, which ever is sooner, should be considered. Neonatal ophthalmic examination should be organised at birth. If the infection occurs after 20 weeks there is still a risk of maternal varicella pneumonia.

If the pregnant woman is in the second half of pregnancy and is seen less than 24 hours after the development of a varicella rash then aciclovir may be expected to reduce the severity and duration of the illness. There are theoretical concerns about teratogenesis when aciclovir is used in the first trimester but these have not been confirmed. Delay of delivery by 5–7 days after the onset of maternal illness allows for the passive transfer of antibodies.

1.30 ADE

Primary amenorrhoea can be due to several causes:

- Constitutional/idiopathic – this accounts for about 15% of the cases. In these instances the gonadotrophins are usually low.
- Gonadal failure – includes pure gonadal dysgenesis, Turner syndrome and non-dysgenetic failure. Serum gonadotrophins are raised and this occurs in about 45% of cases.
- Hypothalamic pituitary dysfunction, such as hypogonadotrophic hypogonadism (Kallmann's syndrome) – in these instances the serum gonadotrophins are low; they account for about 25% of the cause of delayed puberty.
- Defective steroid synthesis – this can cause primary amenorrhoea and delayed puberty as well as chronic illnesses and malnutrition. In both these instances gonadotrophin concentrations are low.

Causes of secondary amenorrhoea are:

- Physiological causes – pregnancy, menopause.
- Gonadotrophin abnormalities – hyperprolactinaemia, structural problems in the pituitary, hypogonadotrophic hypogonadism, polycystic ovarian syndrome, weight loss, chronic illness and psychogenic causes.
- Primary ovarian failure, premature menopause, resistant ovarian syndrome, genital tract abnormalities, eg Asherman syndrome, and other endocrinopathies, eg thyroid dysfunction (hypothyroidism).

1.31 ACD

The incidence of various diseases is different in African women. In incidence of fibroids is increased, although endometriosis is relatively rare. Ectopic pregnancy does seem to be increased, but this is probably associated with tubal disease following pelvic inflammatory disease. Postmenopausal osteoporosis is less common.

1.32 ADE

Clomifene citrate has oestrogenic and anti-oestrogenic properties. It should not be given to women who are ovulating because it will interfere with the oestradiol receptors in the endometrium, raise basal luteinising hormone and possibly affect the production of cervical mucus. Sometimes human chorionic gonadotrophin can be given along with clomiphene to induce ovulation. Human menopausal gonadotrophin is a mixture of follicle-stimulating hormone and luteinising hormone which acts mainly on follicular growth. Ovum release and luteinisation can then be achieved by use of human chorionic gonadotrophin.

1.33 BE

All women with threatened abortion do not need anti-D as some may not be rhesus negative. There is no indication for giving anti-D during an in vitro fertilisation cycle. Even in rhesus-negative women, anti-D is no longer necessary in women with threatened miscarriage unless there is a large amount of vaginal bleeding.

1.34 AD

The progestogen-only pill is less effective than the combined pill but there are no serious adverse effects. The dose of progestogen is much lower than that in the combined pill. The newer desogestrel pill does cause anovulation and is claimed to be as effective as the combined contraceptive pill.

1.35 BCD

The Collaborative Eclampsia Trial found that women treated with magnesium sulphate have fewer recurrent seizures compared with women treated with diazepam or phenytoin. It seems to reduce cerebral vasospasm. Treatment is monitored by hourly measurement of the patellar reflex and respiratory rate or oxygen saturation. If reflexes are absent then magnesium should be discontinued until their return. Respiratory depression should be treated with calcium gluconate.

1.36 BCDE

A painful tender calf is suspicious of a deep vein thrombosis that may be associated with a pulmonary embolism. The signs and symptoms of pulmonary embolism can easily be missed. Typically, there is a pleuritic pain associated with haemoptysis, dyspnoea and, in severe cases, hypertension. Other suspicious features include a dry cough, pyrexia and tachycardia.

1.37 CDE

The table below shows the Royal College of Obstetricians and Gynaecologists, Scientific Advisory Committee, advice on preventing thromboembolism in pregnant women travelling by air.

Any gestation and up to 6 weeks' post partum	Short-haul flight (up to 4 hours)	Long-haul flight (4 hours or more)
No additional risk factors	Calf exercise; move around cabin; avoid dehydration; minimise alcohol and coffee consumption	Calf exercise; move around cabin; avoid dehydration; minimise alcohol and coffee consumption; well-fitting elastic compression stockings
Additional risk factors* Weight ≥ 100 kg or body mass index (BMI) at booking ≥ 30+ Multiple pregnancy Thrombophilia Past personal or strong family history Medical disorders with increased risk of deep vein thrombosis	Calf exercise; move around cabin; avoid dehydration; minimise alcohol and coffee consumption; well-fitting elastic below-knee compression stockings	Calf exercise; move around cabin; avoid dehydration; minimise alcohol and coffee consumption; well-fitting elastic below-knee compression stockings; low-molecular-weight heparin† on day of travel (pre-flight) and day after

*Women with additional risk factors may need to seek appropriate medical advice; some, for instance will already be on thrombo-prophylactic medication.

†Thrombo-prophylactic doses are 5000 units dalteparin or 40 mg enoxaparin. (Low-dose aspirin (75 mg/day for 3 days before travel and on day of travel) is an acceptable alternative in those unable to take low-molecular-weight heparin.)

1.38 BE

The main causes of infertility are shown below. Remember that some couples may have more than one cause.

- Unexplained – 30%
- Sperm defects – 25%
- Ovulatory failure – 20%
- Tubal damage – 15%
- Others – 10%
- Endometriosis – 5%
- Mucus defects – 5%
- Other male problems – 2%
- Coital failure – 2%

1.39 ABC

Fits may be associated with a range of problems, including:

- hypoglycaemia
- birth trauma
- asphyxia
- congenital structural abnormalities of the brain
- meningitis.

1.40 ABCD

A semen sample should be collected after a minimum of 3 days and a maximum of 5 days' abstinence. The sample should be brought to the laboratory within an hour of production and examined as soon as possible. Normal semen variables are:

- Volume > 2–6 ml
- Density > 20 × 10^6/ml
- Motility > 40% forward progression after 2 hours
- Morphology > 20% normal
- White blood cells <1 × 10^6 ml

1.41 BCD

Hyperprolactinaemia is associated with anovulation. Raised serum prolactin interferes with the hypothalamic release of gonadotrophin-releasing hormone. Hyperprolactinaemia may be due to an adenoma of the pituitary or may possibly be related to drugs, especially the phenothiazines. Women with polycystic ovarian syndrome may present with infrequent periods or no periods at all. They are often, but not always, obese with hirsutism and acne. Strenuous exercise or excessive weight loss may suggest a hypothalamic cause with a history of amenorrhoea. Wedge resection used to be a treatment for polycystic ovarian syndrome. Electrodiathermy is gaining acceptance as a treatment for polycystic ovarian infertility.

1.42 AD

Endometriosis is the presence of functional endometrial tissue outside the uterine cavity; it can also occur outside the pelvic cavity (it can occur in the umbilicus or even in abdominal scars). Ideally, histological examination of deposits is not essential for clinical diagnosis. Histological diagnosis is only in retrospect for adenomyosis. Adenomyosis occurs when endometrial tissue lies within the myometrium and is thus a histological diagnosis that can only be made at hysterectomy. Incidence of endometriosis seems to be increasing in general. The incidence also increases with age, with a peak around 40–45 years. About 10% of menstruating Caucasian women have endometriosis. They may be asymptomatic or may have marked symptoms. It is interesting that the extent of the disease is not correlated to the symptoms. Endometriosis is associated with infertility but may not always be so. Endometriosis can cause anatomical distortion and this usually occurs in severe cases. Mild endometriosis with peritoneal deposits may upset fertilisation and there is now evidence that ablating these areas may be beneficial – drug treatment does not improve conception rates.

1.43 ABD

Primary cytomegalovirus (CMV) infection during pregnancy may affect both the placenta and the fetus in up to 50% of cases. The prognosis of the infection in the fetus is not accurately known, but it may produce microcephaly, choroidoretinitis, eighth nerve damage, pneumonia, hepatosplenomegaly, anaemia (sometimes haemolytic with jaundice) and intrauterine growth retardation. Myocarditis and enterocolitis are not usually associated with CMV infection.

1.44 BCD

The following patients are most likely to request reversal of sterilisation:

- A patient who was sterilised before the age of 30
- A patient who is in an unstable relationship
- A patient from a lower socioeconomic class
- A woman who was sterilised immediately after a pregnancy or during a termination of pregnancy
- A patient who has neurotic traits

Up to 60% of women requesting reversal of sterilisation want children by another partner. The rate of success does depend on the method of sterilisation and reversal of clip sterilisation is easier than that following diathermy to the tubes. The ectopic rate after any reversal of sterilisation is about 3%. Most surgeons find that magnification helps and use of an operating microscope is ideal. Raised levels of follicle-stimulating hormone indicate ovarian malfunction and reduced fertility. It needs to be repeated and then counselling should be offered – reversal may not be appropriate. Do not forget to discuss in vitro fertilisation as an alternative.

1.45 CD

Laparoscopy is now being used more and more and contraindications are decreasing. Chronic tuberculous peritonitis is a contraindication because this is associated with quite marked abdominal adhesions and perforation of the bowel may go unrecognised. However, other previous abdominal surgery is not a contraindication. A laparoscopy is a regular method of detecting an ectopic pregnancy and is not, therefore, contraindicated in a pregnancy. In the advanced stages of pregnancy it is obviously contraindicated because of the damage that may occur.

1.46 BDE

Physiological jaundice in a healthy baby appears after the first 48 hours of life, reaches a peak by about the fourth day and disappears within 7–10 days. The bowel is usually sterile at birth but is rapidly colonised by organisms that include those encountered along the birth canal and perineum. Urine is passed *in utero* as can be seen on ultrasound and is often passed at or soon after birth. The respiratory rate is usually less than 60/min at rest, 25–35 being usual. Constriction of the ductus arteriosus occurs because of the direct effect on the vessel wall of raising the arteriolar oxygen pressure with ventilation of the lungs at birth. There is probably a rapid partial closure soon after birth followed by a more gradual closure during the course of several days.

1.47 AC

Obesity is associated with an increased level of unopposed oestrogens. Endometrial carcinoma is usually an adenocarcinoma and a negative cervical smear does not exclude it. The smear may pick up abnormal endometrial cells. Unopposed oestrogen stimulation, either endogenous or exogenous, is associated with endometrial carcinoma. There is a 6% risk of this after five years of unopposed oral oestrogens. The addition of a progestogen reduces the incidence to a relative risk of 0.9.

1.48 ACE

Maternal height is of limited value in predicting fetopelvic disproportion, although the rate of caesarean section tends to be higher among short mothers. Because of the large overlap in the obstetrical outcome between women with small and large dimensions, the statistical significance of correlations between maternal height or shoe size and cephalopelvic disproportion is limited. Non-engagement of the head may be associated with cephalopelvic disproportion in primigravidae, but it is not diagnostic. The role of X-ray pelvimetry is limited – neither X-ray nor clinical pelvimetry has been shown to predict cephalopelvic disproportion with sufficient accuracy to justify elective caesarean section for cephalic presentation. Cephalopelvic disproportion is best diagnosed by carefully monitoring the trial of labour, and X-ray pelvimetry should seldom, if ever, be necessary.

1.49 BC

Polyhydramnios (increased liquor volume) is associated with failure of reabsorption of liquor or an increase in production. This occurs in oesophageal atresia and open neural tube defects. Ovarian hyperstimulation syndrome causes ascites but not polyhydramnios. Potter syndrome is associated with renal agenesis and this leads to oligo rather than polyhydramnios.

1.50 D

Preterm or premature birth is defined by the World Health Organization as delivery of an infant before 37 completed weeks' of gestation. There is no set lower limit. It occurs in about 5–10% of births. Causes of preterm births are:

- unexplained – 30% (risk factors include: low socioeconomic group and previous preterm labour)
- genital tract infection
- preterm premature rupture of membranes
- multiple pregnancy (30%)
- antepartum haemorrhage
- cervical incompetence
- congenital uterine abnormalities
- elective (intrauterine growth retardation congenital abnormalities medical disorders).

About 70% of preterm labours progress to delivery.

1.51 DE

Bacterial vaginosis is associated with the following complications of pregnancy:

- Low birth weight
- Preterm labour
- Preterm birth
- Premature rupture of membranes
- Late miscarriage
- Chorioamnionitis
- Endometritis after caesarean section

There is evidence that anti-anaerobic treatment may reduce chances of other premature deliveries.

1.52 CDE

At booking it is important that the individual woman is assessed. Risks and needs need to be dealt with and the antenatal care should be adapted to their own particular requirements. Seat belts must be worn in the correct fashion. As part of the full risk assessment, the body mass index should be calculated. Women then should be advised about sensible weight reduction, including diet and exercise, and referral to a dietitian where appropriate.

A full psychiatric history is important. The term postnatal depression should only be used to describe a non-psychotic depressive illness of mild to moderate severity with its onset following delivery. Suggested reading: *Why Mothers Die 1997–1999* (CEMACH).

1.53 BC

The effectiveness of advice given during pregnancy has to be questioned and evaluated as rigorously as any other intervention in medicine and pregnancy. Advice about sexual activity is conflicting. Published evidence suggests that prevention of sexual activity during pregnancy is inappropriate. However, there is strong evidence that maternal smoking reduces birth weight and that excessive alcohol consumption causes fetal damage. Excessive alcohol consumption is associated with fetal growth retardation, learning disabilities and altered neonatal behaviour. There does not seem to be any scientific evidence that supports decreasing work, indeed, stopping work may actually increase the amount of housework that one does and also lead to financial stress. Folic acid in a dose of 0.4 mg/day is now advised with 5 mg/day for women who have already had a baby with spina bifida. The folic acid supplementation should start 3 months before conception and continue until 12 weeks' gestation.

1.54 BCE

The most common bacteria that cause PID are *Chlamydia trachomatis* and *Neisseria gonorrhoeae*. These cause damage to the epithelial surface, following which opportunist organisms, including *Mycoplasma hominis* and anaerobes, invade. PID is associated with high morbidity, including:

- 20% women become infertile
- 20% women develop chronic pelvic pain
- 10% of those who conceive have an ectopic pregnancy.

Factors associated with PID mirror those for sexually transmitted infections including:

- Young age
- lower socioeconomic status
- African/African Caribbean ethnicity
- Lower educational attainment
- Recent ascending infection

1.55 DE

An understanding the physiological anaemia of pregnancy is important and there is evidence that what seems to be a low haemoglobin may be beneficial in pregnancy. Few randomised trials have monitored the effects of giving iron supplementation as a matter of routine, but it does not have any beneficial effects on proteinuria, hypertension, antepartum haemorrhage or maternal infection. Anaemia may actually be detrimental to the outcome of pregnancy as a few well-conducted trials have shown that preterm delivery and low birth weight are increased. The associated pathology may be increased blood viscosity following the iron-induced macrocytosis and thus an impedance to utero-placental blood flow.

1.56 ACD

OHSS is an iatrogenic potentially life-threatening condition resulting from excessive ovarian induction treatment. The pathophysiology of this syndrome is not clearly understood. The treatment of OHSS is often careful observation (mild or moderate OHSS). Some women (severe OHSS) require hospitalisation and supportive treatment. In mild OHSS, the woman may complain of mild abdominal discomfort and the ovaries are usually less than 5 cm in diameter. Moderate OHSS results in more noticeable pain and vomiting, and the ovaries measure between 5 cm and 10 cm. In the severe form, the ovaries are > 10 cm in diameter and there is free intraperitoneal fluid, pleural effusions, hypotension and oliguria. If no pregnancy occurs, the syndrome will typically resolve within a week. In the setting of a maintained pregnancy, slow resolution of symptoms usually occurs over 1–2 months. The prevalence of mild and moderate forms of OHSS has been reported as between 10% and 20% in all women undergoing ovulation induction treatment and the use of gonadotrophins. Severe forms of OHSS occur in < 1% of women undergoing ovulation induction.

1.57 AD

The postnatal blues are a brief period of emotional distress which can occur between the third and the tenth day postpartum. It is a common condition and occurs in 50–80% of all women who give birth. The blues are characterised by tearfulness, irritability and distress.

Postnatal psychosis is a rare and more dramatic disorder that affects 0.2% of women in the postpartum period. Symptoms may occur within the first 6 weeks after delivery and include marked disturbance in mood characterised by a very high or elated mood or a very low, depressed mood and a disturbance in perception in which auditory or visual hallucinations can occur as well as behaviour disturbances. A woman experiencing postpartum psychosis is very much at risk, and her infant and other children may also be in danger. She must be referred to a psychiatrist immediately.

If a mother develops postnatal psychosis she has a 1 in 5 chance of developing it again in the next pregnancy.

1.58 D

The normal fetal heart rate (FHR) pattern is characterised by a baseline frequency between 110 and 150 beats per minute, presence of periodic accelerations, a normal heart rate variability between 5 and 25 beats per minute and the absence of decelerations. Recording speeds vary from 1–3 cm per minute. β-mimetics, such as ritodrine, increase the baseline FHR and are associated with a decrease in FHR variability. Magnesium sulphate causes a decrease in FHR variability. Most cases of cerebral palsy have antecedents in the antenatal period, with only about 10% of cases having an intrapartum cause.

1.59 ACE

The menopause is the permanent cessation of menstruation resulting from loss of ovarian follicular activity. Natural menopause is recognised to have occurred after 12 consecutive months of amenorrhoea for which there is no obvious pathological or physiological cause. Menopause occurs with the final period and is only known with certainty in retrospect. Premature menopause is defined as menopause that occurs at an age less than two standard deviations below the mean for the reference population. In the developed world this is considered to be 40 years.

1.60 None

It is interesting that blood loss can be influenced by many factors, including emotional upsets, marital problems or even a fear of genital cancer. It is important to take a good history and it is true to say that, although a history may be unreliable, most women would not generally wish to have a gynaecological examination without good reason and, thus, the complaint must commonly be assumed to be a real complaint. Clip sterilisations are not associated with heavy periods. Before rushing into a major surgical procedure, medical treatment and even more minor surgical procedures would be the first line of treatment. Abnormal menstrual bleeding may be ovulatory or anovulatory in origin. As a rule of thumb, irregular, prolonged cycles are associated with anovulation and regular cycles are associated with ovulation and structural deformities. Anovulation is more common around puberty and the climacteric and about 20% of women who present with menstrual dysfunction will have anovulatory cycles.

EXTENDED MATCHING QUESTIONS ANSWERS

THEME: MINOR DISORDERS OF PREGNANCY

1.61 C Antacids are indicated for the initial management. Proton pump inhibitors are rarely used for this indication.

1.62 E Explanation and reassurance. Analgesics are not used for this indication as they are not usually effective. Explanation and reassurance are all that is needed. Expert advice from an obstetric physiotherapist is useful in more severe cases.

1.63 F Dietary fibre is needed, lubricant laxatives may be harmful.

THEME: GENITAL TRACT INFECTIONS

1.64 G *Trichomonas vaginalis* presents with such a typical picture.

1.65 A *Chlamydia trachomatis* causes severe tubal damage.

1.66 C *Haemophilus ducreyi* causes a typical soft chancre, usually on the vulva.

Questions on pages 29–38

THEME: DEEP VENOUS THROMBOSIS IN PREGNANCY

1.67 C Low-molecular-weight heparin – subcutaneous. Initial management includes starting treatment for the thrombosis until the diagnosis is excluded (or confirmed) by objective testing. Low-molecular-weight heparin is more effective and associated with less risk of haemorrhage and lower mortality than unfractionated heparin.

1.68 C Low-molecular-weight heparin – subcutaneous. Therapeutic doses of low-molecular-weight heparin are indicated for maintenance treatment. Warfarin crosses the placenta and can cause embryopathy, central nervous system abnormalities and fetal haemorrhage. Prolonged use of unfractionated heparin can cause osteoporosis and fractures.

1.69 E Unfractionated heparin, given intravenously has a short half-life and therefore can be stopped and the effects reversed in the event of a haemorrhage.

THEME: PRESCRIBING FOR BREAST-FEEDING WOMEN

1.70 F Fluoxetine is secreted in the breast milk but effects do not warrant stopping feeding or withholding the drug.

1.71 C Treatment with a broad-spectrum antibiotic is indicated. Co-amoxiclav is safe for breast-feeding women.

1.72 H Warfarin can be used in breast-feeding women.

THEME: SUBFERTILITY

1.73 C A laparoscopy and dye test would allow the assessment of pelvic organs, and tubal patency can be evaluated at the same time.

1.74 F Semen analysis. A sperm count would avoid unnecessary invasive tests on the woman and is a simple test that can exclude male factor infertility.

1.75 A Hormone profiles. The history points towards polycystic ovary syndrome, hence a hormone profile would aid the diagnosis.

THEME: PRETERM LABOUR

1.76 B Atosiban is a licensed drug for the suppression of preterm labour. Nifedipine is an unlicensed alternative. Neither ritodrine or magnesium sulphate is recommended by the Royal College of Obstetricians and Gynaecologists for this indication.

1.77 D Caesarean section. The cervix is too dilated for successful suppression and the footling breech presentation would usually warrant caesarean section because of the risk of prolapsed cord and delivery through an incompletely dilated cervix.

1.78 A Labour suppression is often not successful with ruptured membranes.

THEME: UTEROVAGINAL PROLAPSE

1.79 B Cystocele. The bulge is the bladder base due to lax anterior vaginal wall muscles.

1.80 D Rectocele. This is rectal prolapse through lax posterior vaginal wall muscles.

1.81 C Enterocele. Occasionally small bowel can prolapse through a weakness in the posterior vaginal fornix.

THEME: URINARY INCONTINENCE

1.82 A Detrusor overactivity.

1.83 C This is possibly a vesicovaginal fistula that is typical of the history given.

1.84 G Urodynamic stress incontinence.

THEME: PERINATAL STATISTICS

1.85 A < 10%

1.86 D 50–60%

1.87 F > 90%

THEME: ABDOMINAL PAIN

1.88 B Fibroid degeneration. Fibroids are common in women of African Caribbean origin. They are associated with heavy periods and undergo degeneration, associated with acute lower abdominal pains and vomiting.

1.89 G Primary dysmenorrhoea typically presents in young girls at the beginning of their reproductive lives and the pain precedes menstrual flow.

1.90 D This is a classic presentation of ovarian hyperstimulation syndrome – with a history of fertility treatment and lower abdominal pains associated with vomiting.

Practice Paper 2 Questions

BEST OF FIVE QUESTIONS

20 Questions: Time allowed 30 minutes. Please give the single most appropriate answer from the list of alternatives.

2.1 In which one of these fetal conditions is termination of pregnancy not justified?

- A Anencephaly
- B Triploidy
- C Trisomy 18
- D Gastroschisis
- E Bilateral renal agenesis

2.2 A 28-year-old woman has received her triple test (maternal serum screen analysing three markers) result as part of a screening programme for Down syndrome. The result is 1 in 100. Which one of the following is the most likely course of action?

- A Request a repeat triple test
- B Request an amniocentesis
- C Refuse any further tests because she is low risk as she is only 28
- D Request a chorion villus sample (CVS)
- E Request a termination of pregnancy

Answers on pages 113–117

2.3 Which one of the following statements is not appropriate with regard to drug use in pregnancy?

A The fetus is most vulnerable to drug teratogenicity at 2–8 weeks

B Diethylstilbestrol use can be associated with clear cell adenocarcinoma in female offspring

C Isotretinoin is associated with multiple abnormalities

D Phenothiazines are associated with Ebstein anomaly

E There are no randomised studies on the safety of drugs in pregnancy

2.4 You are attending a couple with subfertility. The male partner has subnormal sperm counts. With regard to male subfertility, with which one of the following statements do you agree?

A There is little variability in sperm quality when assessed in the same individual over time

B Use of gonadotrophin drugs in hypogonadotropic hypogonadal men is not an effective treatment

C Steroids are an effective treatment for antisperm antibodies

D Following reversal of vasectomy there is an 80% chance of a subsequent pregnancy

E Varicocele surgery improves the rate of pregnancy in most oligozoospermic men

2.5 A woman is admitted with lower abdominal pain and 8 weeks amenorrhoea followed by vaginal bleeding. An ectopic pregnancy is suspected. Which one of the following factors would decrease the suspicion of an ectopic pregnancy?

- A Intrauterine contraceptive device (IUCD) failure
- B Passage of small pieces of tissue vaginally
- C Previous abdominal surgery
- D A history of multiple sexual partners
- E Previous infertility

2.6 A pregnant woman has been found to have *Chlamydia trachomatis* infection. She asks you about the infection. Which one of the following statements is true?

- A The infection affects about 25% women attending at general practices
- B 50% of the women are asymptomatic
- C The infection can be transmitted to the neonate at the time of delivery
- D Contact tracing is not necessary
- E Ampicillin 1 gm single dose is an effective treatment

2.7 In which one of the following circumstances should cervical screening be performed routinely?

- A Screening sexually active teenagers is justifiable
- B Screening should never cease in old age
- C Screening should begin at 25 years of age
- D All women should be tested annually
- E Screening is not possible at a 6-week postnatal check

2.8 An older woman complains of urinary incontinence. Which one of the following symptoms is suggestive of detrusor instability?

- A Dysuria
- B Constipation leading to faecal impaction
- C Urge incontinence
- D Haematuria
- E Dribbling following micturition

2.9 A 75-year-old woman is being treated for a urinary tract infection (UTI). Which one of the following is the most likely feature of the problem?

- A Females are less prone to UTI than males
- B Significant bacteriuria represents a bacterial count > 10 000 CFU/ml
- C Asymptomatic bacteriuria affects approximately 30% of older women
- D Oral oestrogen treatment reduces recurrent UTI in postmenopausal women
- E Nitrofurantoin is unsafe for treating UTI
- F Sulphonamides are unsafe for treating UTI

2.10 An anxious primigravida requests an induction of labour without admission to hospital. Which one of the following is a recommended method for induction of labour?

- A Sexual intercourse
- B Nipple stimulation
- C Acupuncture
- D Castor oil
- E 'Stretch and sweep'

2.11 In a primigravida with severe pre-eclampsia (blood pressure 170/11 mmHg, 4+ proteinuria), which one of the following symptoms/signs is most likely to indicate imminent eclampsia?

- A Severe chest pain
- B Vomiting
- C Visual disturbances
- D Pedal oedema
- E Anuria

2.12 With regard to termination of pregnancy which one of the following statements is appropriate?

- A In the UK, the law allows a woman to have an abortion up to a limit of 20 weeks of pregnancy if two doctors agree that it would cause less damage to her physical and mental health than continuing the pregnancy
- B A woman should not wait for > 3 weeks from first referral to the time of termination
- C A girl < 16 years old cannot consent for termination if the pregnancy is > 8 weeks
- D *Chlamydia* testing should not be routinely performed before termination
- E Suction termination is best performed after 4 weeks of pregnancy

2.13 It is important to explain to women all the risks associated an operation. Which one of the following need not be mentioned with regard to a day case laparoscopic tubal occlusion?

A Failure rate of 1:200

B Risk of ectopic pregnancy if failure occurs

C Uterine perforation

D Risk of deep vein thrombosis

E Risk of laparotomy

2.14 When caring for a terminally ill cancer patient, which one of the following is justified?

A Radiotherapy is not used to relieve pain in specific instances such as bony metastasis

B Diarrhoea occurs initially but later settles with use of morphine

C Tricyclic antidepressants are not effective in neuropathic pain

D Corticosteroids should never be used because of the risk of osteoporosis

E Transcutaneous electrical nerve stimulation (TENS) can be sometimes used for relief

2.15 A woman comes into contact with a case of chicken pox when she is in the first trimester of pregnancy. Which one of the following is the most appropriate first step in her management?

A Offer termination of pregnancy

B Prescribe aciclovir

C Check her immunity with varicella zoster IgG titre

D Prescribe immunoglobulin

E Perform an ultrasound examination of the fetus

2.16 With regard to pregnancy in rhesus-negative women and anti-D prophylaxis, which one of the following statements is appropriate?

A About 0.3% of women have feto-maternal haemorrhage > 15 ml

B Up to 5% of greater feto-maternal haemorrhage occurs after delivery

C Anti-D should be given to all women with spontaneous miscarriage before 12 weeks of pregnancy

D Anti-D should be given to sensitised anti-D negative women after amniocentesis

E At least 500 IU of anti-D should be given to non-sensitised rhesus-negative women at 20 and 30 weeks prophylactically

2.17 With regard to the management of a woman with pelvic inflammatory disease (PID), which one of the following represents the best management option?

- A Laparoscopy must be performed in all cases.
- B Ofloxacin is safe to be given to young women.
- C Intrauterine contraceptive device (IUCD) should be removed in all cases of severe PID
- D Women with PID in pregnancy do not usually need treatment
- E Treatment for PID should not be undertaken in the outpatient clinic

2.18 You and your registrar are called by a midwife to perform an operative vaginal delivery for delay in the second stage of labour. The fetal head is 0/5ths palpable abdominally, membranes are ruptured, bladder is empty and there is a working epidural. The position is left-occipito-transverse, no caput or moulding. Which one of the following is the most likely course of action?

- A Vacuum extraction
- B Neville–Barnes (non-rotational) forceps delivery
- C Caesarean section
- D Do nothing and wait
- E Wrigley (lift out) forceps delivery

2.19 When considering prophylaxis for venous thromboembolism in the puerperium which one factor does not constitute an increase in risk?

- A Age > 35 years
- B Body mass index > 30 kg/m^2
- C Parity > 4
- D Emergency caesarean section
- E Outlet instrumental delivery

2.20 When counselling a woman about exercise in pregnancy which one of the following statements represents the most appropriate advice?

- A Adverse pregnancy or neonatal outcomes are increased in exercising women
- B Initiating pelvic floor exercises in postpartum period may reduce risk of future urinary incontinence
- C Weight-bearing exercise throughout pregnancy can increase the length of labour
- D Exercise in supine position is not a problem after 16 weeks of pregnancy
- E Scuba diving and horse riding could be continued during pregnancy

MULTIPLE CHOICE QUESTIONS

40 Questions: Time allowed 1½ hours. Indicate your answers clearly by putting a tick against the correct or true options and a cross against the incorrect or false options. (The section on answers in this book lists the correct (true) options.)

2.21 There is a recognisable chromosome abnormality in which of the following syndromes?

- A Klinefelter syndrome
- B Tay–Sachs disease
- C Achondroplasia
- D Cri-du-chat syndrome
- E Patau syndrome

2.22 Endometriosis can be treated with:

- A Medroxyprogesterone acetate
- B Danazol
- C Evening primrose oil
- D Mefenamic acid
- E Luteinising hormone releasing hormone analogues

Answers on pages 119–139

2.23 An oblique lie:

A May be transitory

B Usually turns to a longitudinal lie

C After 33 weeks needs to be admitted to hospital due to the risk of cord prolapse

D Should be treated by external cephalic version (ECV) at 37 weeks

E Is associated with placenta praevia

2.24 With regard to breech presentation:

A At 28 weeks the incidence of breech presentation is 40%

B The incidence of breech presentation at term is 3–4%

C The perinatal mortality and morbidity with breech presentations is the same as with vertex

D All women with uncomplicated breech pregnancy at term (37–42 weeks) should be offered external cephalic version

E The best method of delivering a term frank or complete breech singleton is by planned caesarean section

2.25 Renal changes typical of a normal pregnancy include:

A Increased glomerular filtration rate

B Decreased excretion of urate

C Increased excretion of folate

D Increased excretion of glucose

E Ureteric dilatation

2.26 Pruritus vulvae may be associated with:

A Diabetes

B Raynaud disease

C Threadworm infection

D Thyroid disease

E Renal failure

2.27 Pregnancy is associated with:

A Increase in cardiac output

B Decrease in central venous pressure

C Increase in peripheral resistance

D Increase in pulse rate

E Decrease in stroke volume

2.28 Depo-Provera:

A Is the most widely used form of injectable contraception

B Can effect lactation

C Has a failure rate ranging from 5 to 7 pregnancies/100 women years

D In adequate doses suppresses ovulation

E Has no effect on cervical mucus

2.29 Which of the following definitions is/are correct?

A A late death is a death occurring between 42 days and 1 year after abortion or delivery that is due to direct or indirect maternal causes

B A stillbirth is the birth, after 24 weeks' gestation, of an infant who does not show signs of life

C Perinatal mortality is defined as stillbirths plus first-week neonatal deaths expressed per 1000 total births

D Neonatal death is a live-born infant who dies within 28 days of birth (whatever gestation if signs of life are noted)

E Maternities is a count of the number of mothers delivered of live or stillborn infants as distinct from the number of babies born, which includes twins and other multiple births

2.30 With regard to endometriosis:

A It occurs with increasing age

B It has a peak incidence between the ages of 50 and 55

C It occurs in about 1% of Caucasians

D The extent of the disease correlates well with the symptoms

E It may be a normal clinical finding

2.31 Non-sensitised rhesus-negative women should receive anti-D immunoglobulin in which of the following situations?

- A Ectopic pregnancy after 12 weeks
- B Any miscarriage after 8 weeks
- C All miscarriages in which surgical evacuation is performed
- D All miscarriages in which medical evacuation is performed
- E Any threatened miscarriage when there is heavy vaginal bleeding or associated abdominal pain

2.32 Medical treatment of dysfunctional uterine bleeding includes:

- A Oral contraceptives
- B Mefenamic acid
- C Cyclical progestogens
- D Cyclical oestrogens
- E Evening primrose oil

2.33 With regard to cervical smears:

- A A negative result excludes frank carcinoma
- B Persistent inflammatory results warrant colposcopic examination
- C Koilocytosis is suggestive of human papillomavirus (HPV) infection
- D Dyskaryosis is caused by *Trichomonas vaginalis*
- E They are best performed postnatally at 6 weeks

2.34 Management of a pregnant woman who presents with chickenpox includes:

A Isolation from all other pregnant women and neonates

B Delivery ideally should be delayed until 5–7 days after the onset of maternal illness

C If delivery occurs within 5 days of maternal infection, then the neonate should be given varicella zoster immunoglobulin (VZIG) as soon as possible

D Varicella pneumonia is an indication for treatment with intravenous aciclovir

E Where maternal infection occurs 5 days before or 2 days after delivery there is a 20–30% risk of varicella of the newborn

2.35 With regard to miscarriage:

A Miscarriage is known to occur in 3% of clinical pregnancies

B In a threatened miscarriage bedrest should be encouraged

C Medical management is not an acceptable method in the management of confirmed miscarriage

D Risks of surgical evacuation include intra-abdominal trauma

E If a woman is undergoing surgical evacuation she should be screened for *Chlamydia trachomatis*

2.36 With regard to gestational age of a newborn baby:

A At 36 weeks of age the ear returns to its shape after folding

B At 38 weeks of age there is no palpable breast tissue

C At 38 weeks of age the testes have few scrotal rugae

D At 40 weeks of age there is good arm recoil after extension at the elbow

E At 40 weeks of age the baby is pale pink with slight superficial skin peeling

2.37 With regard to placenta praevia:

A Transvaginal ultrasound is safe in the presence of placenta praevia

B Women with major placenta praevia, as per recent evidence, do not need to be admitted to hospital

C Cervical cerclage should be considered

D Caesarean section is the management of choice for women whose placenta is 10 cm or less from the os

E A hysterectomy may be required to help control haemorrhage at the time of caesarean section

2.38 Endometriosis:

A Occurs in about 20% of women being investigated for infertility

B May present with a pelvic mass

C Can be easily diagnosed by ultrasound scanning

D May be associated with raised levels of CA125

E Is always symptomatic

2.39 Neonatal hypocalcaemia:

- A May be due to maternal dietary deficiency
- B Often accompanies hypoglycaemia
- C May cause permanent brain damage
- D Is a common cause of convulsions
- E Is seen in association with a normal maternal blood calcium concentration

2.40 Polycystic ovarian syndrome (PCOS):

- A Was first described by Stein and Leventhal in 1935
- B Is associated with a low serum luteinising hormone concentration
- C May be associated with anovulation, hirsutism, obesity and reduced ovarian stroma
- D Can be associated with hypoinsulinaemia
- E May be associated with recurrent miscarriages

2.41 With regard to carcinoma of the cervix:

- A It is the commonest malignant cause of female deaths
- B The death rate has been markedly reduced by the British screening programme
- C Most women dying from the condition have never had a smear
- D It has a decreased incidence in smokers
- E The treatment of choice is radiotherapy in the obese woman

2.42 With regard to hormone replacement therapy used in specific medical conditions:

A There is high risk of increasing the size of a fibroid

B It is contraindicated in diabetes mellitus

C It is contraindicated in otosclerosis

D It should be considered in renal failure

E It may increase the risk of gallbladder disease

2.43 In Down syndrome:

A Most people have an extra number 21 chromosome

B Trisomy is usually due to non-disjunction during meiosis

C A female with Down syndrome will never have a normal child

D Women over the age of 40 years have a risk of 1 in 200 of having a child with Down syndrome

E A reduced serum concentration of α-fetoprotein in amniotic fluid may be associated with an affected fetus

2.44 Micro-organisms capable of penetrating the placental barrier and infecting the fetus are:

A *Staphylococcus aureus*

B *Toxoplasma gondii*

C Cytomegalovirus

D Varicella zoster virus

E Hepatitis B virus

2.45 Scabies:

A Is due to infestation by the mite *Sarcoptes scabiei*

B Infestation is after close physical contact

C Symptoms usually occur within 12 hours of infestation

D Treatment is with application of 25% benzyl benzoate

E Itching is usually relieved within 48 hours after successful treatment

2.46 Gestational diabetes:

A Is defined as glucose intolerance appearing during pregnancy

B Is associated with a small increase in perinatal mortality

C Is best treated with insulin

D Is associated with fetal macrosomia

E If treated with insulin, reduces the incidence of fetal macrosomia

2.47 Luteinising hormone releasing hormone (LHRH) analogues are effective in the treatment of:

A Menorrhagia

B Endometriosis

C Uterine fibroids

D Osteoporosis

E Granuloma cell tumour of the ovary

2.48 In the fetus:

- A The umbilical arteries carry oxygenated blood
- B The ductus venosus short circuits the capillaries of the liver
- C The right atrium contains a mixture of oxygenated and venous blood
- D The foramen ovale connects the ventricles of the heart
- E The ductus arteriosus joins the aorta proximal to the aortic arch

2.49 Respiratory distress syndrome of the newborn:

- A Is always obvious at birth when present
- B Causes pathognomonic changes on the chest X-ray
- C Is unusual in full-term babies
- D Responds to supplementation of lung surfactants
- E Should be treated routinely with antibiotics

2.50 Evidence-based treatment options for hyperemesis include:

- A Antihistamines
- B Corticosteroids
- C Phenothiazines
- D Dietary ginger
- E Acupressure

2.51 Genital warts:

A Are benign mesodermal growths on the external perianal and perigenital region

B Caused by the herpes simplex virus

C Are sexually transmitted

D May resolve spontaneously

E Progress to cancer in 3% of cases

2.52 Vulvodynia:

A Is a term used to describe a specific type of vulval pain characterised by burning, stinging, irritation and rawness

B May be caused by vulval eczema

C Can cause dyspareunia

D May be caused by allergy

E Can be treated with local corticosteroids

2.53 Methods that can be used to screen for genetic disease during pregnancy include:

A Ultrasound

B Amniocentesis

C Chorionic villus sampling

D X-ray

E A combination of α-fetoprotein, β-human chorionic gonadotrophin and oestriol levels

2.54 Pelvic inflammatory disease

A Is inflammation of the upper genital tract in women, typically involving the fallopian tubes, ovaries and surrounding structures

B Is best diagnosed by clinical symptoms and signs

C Is always symptomatic

D In most cases is due to an ascending infection from the cervix

E Can be prevented by vaginal douching

2.55 Useful tests for the assessment of fetal well-being in the third trimester are:

A Vaginal ultrasound measurement of crown–rump length

B Human placental lactogen measurement

C Serum α-fetoprotein

D Fetal movement counting

E Amniotic fluid volume measurement

2.56 Women with heart disease in pregnancy:

A With good multidisciplinary care are at no greater risk of maternal death

B Can be given oxytocin in the usual way

C Can present with pyrexia of unknown origin

D Are at additional risk if they have a pulmonary vascular disease

E Should be given careful pre-pregnancy counselling

2.57 Breast-fed children are less likely to have:

A Ear infections (otitis media)

B Allergies

C Vomiting

D Diarrhoea

E Pneumonia, wheezing and bronchiolitis

2.58 Oblique lie is associated with:

A Multiparity

B Uterine abnormalities

C Fundal placenta

D Pelvic tumours

E Small pelvic inlet

2.59 With regard to the menopause:

A Age of the menopause may be determined in utero

B It occurs earlier in women with Down syndrome

C It occurs later in smokers

D Japanese race/ethnicity may be associated with later age of natural menopause

E It results in a fall of oestrogen production

2.60 Ovarian hyperstimulation syndrome (OHSS):

- A Is a complication of induction of ovulation
- B Usually occurs after human chorionic gonadotrophin has been given
- C Is associated with polycystic ovarian syndrome
- D Is associated with a predisposition to thrombosis
- E Can be fatal

EXTENDED MATCHING QUESTIONS

30 Questions: Time allowed 1 hour.

THEME: PRE-PREGNANCY COUNSELLING – RECURRENCE RISKS

A < 1%
B 1–2%
C 10–15%
D 25%
E 33%
F 50%
G 75%
H 100%

Instructions: From the list above choose the uncorrected recurrence risk in a subsequent pregnancy for the occurrence of the following complications. Each option can be used once, more than once or not at all.

2.61 Pre-eclampsia in the first pregnancy.

2.62 Abruptio placenta.

2.63 Impacted shoulders.

Answers on pages 141–145

THEME: EARLY PREGNANCY PROBLEMS

A Antibiotic treatment
B Evacuation of uterus
C Intramuscular human chorionic gonadotrophin (hCG) injections
D Laparoscopy
E Reassurance
F Repeat ultrasound and serum hCG estimation
G Repeat ultrasound of the uterus in 1 week
H Serum hCG estimation
I Conservative management

Instructions: From the list above choose the most appropriate management for each clinical scenario described below. Each option can be used once, more than once or not at all.

2.64 A primiparous woman with a history of 7 weeks' amenorrhoea, vaginal bleeding, pelvic pain and an empty uterus on ultrasound scan.

2.65 A 8-week pregnant woman with pain, passage of clots vaginally and an open cervix on pelvic examination.

2.66 At 7 weeks of amenorrhoea there is ultrasound evidence of a sac present in utero but a fetal heart is not seen.

THEME: GENERAL GYNAECOLOGY

A A 6-month course of gonadotrophin releasing hormone (GnRH) analogues
B Cervical biopsy
C Combined oral contraceptive
D Copper intrauterine contraceptive device (IUCD)
E Endometrial biopsy
F Mirena intrauterine system (IUS)
G Mefenamic acid

Instructions: From the list above choose the most appropriate management plan for the gynaecological scenarios given below. Each option can be used once, more than once or not at all.

2.67 A 33-year-old woman with a fibroid uterus who desires fertility in 8 months' time.

2.68 A 45-year-old woman presents with heavy regular periods for 12 months.

2.69 A 14-year-old girl presents with menorrhagia.

THEME: HORMONE REPLACEMENT THERAPY (HRT)

A Calcium supplements
B Continue HRT
C Do a thrombophilia screen
D Give nothing
E HRT is contraindicated
F HRT is indicated
G Stop HRT
H Sun bathing

Instructions: Regarding use of HRT in different situations choose the most appropriate advice from the list above that you will give to the women presenting in your general practice. Each option can be used once, more than once or not at all.

2.70 A 60-year-old woman with a history of breast cancer has already started taking oestrogen containing HRT.

2.71 A 58-year-old woman comes to ask for advice about HRT. She has a strong family history of deep vein thrombosis and breast cancer in first-degree relatives.

2.72 A 30-year-old woman has premature ovarian failure and is complaining of hot flushes.

THEME: INTRA-UTERINE GROWTH RESTRICTION

A Caesarean section
B Immediate induction of labour
C Induction of labour at term
D Invasive genetic testing
E Routine antenatal care
F Ultrasound for fetal growth
G Umbilical artery Doppler examination

Instructions: From the list above choose the most appropriate management plan for following clinical circumstances. In all cases the fetus is a cephalic presentation and the mother has never had any surgery to the uterus. Each option can be used once, more than once or not at all.

2.73 A primigravida with a clinically small baby at 36 weeks' gestation and an fetal abdominal circumference on the 10th centile (normal umbilical artery Doppler examination).

2.74 An anatomically normal fetus, fetal abdominal circumference on the 5th centile with absent end diastolic flow in the umbilical artery at 34 weeks' gestation.

2.75 A clinically small fetus in a para 2 woman with two normally grown babies.

THEME: VACCINATION IN PREGNANCY

A Administer vaccine if indicated
B Avoid vaccine unless risk of infection is high
C Safe to travel without vaccination
D Travel not recommended
E Unsafe, do not give

Instructions: From the list above choose the most appropriate advice for vaccination in a healthy pregnant woman. Each option can be used once, more than once or not at all.

2.76 Hepatitis B vaccination in a woman who continues the intravenous use of street drugs and is not immune to hepatitis B.

2.77 Rubella vaccination in a woman who is not immune to rubella and who is worried about contracting rubella in this pregnancy.

2.78 Hepatitis A vaccination in a woman travelling to a developing country where there is a risk of hepatitis A.

THEME: MENSTRUAL DISORDERS

A Delayed puberty
B Haematocolpos
C Precocious puberty
D Premature ovarian failure
E Primary amenorrhoea
F Sexual abuse
G Turner syndrome

Instructions: From the list above choose the most appropriate pathology for the menstrual complaints in the following scenarios. Each option can be used once, more than once or not at all.

2.79 A 25-year-old woman presents with hot flushes, amenorrhoea for 8 months and a similar history in her siblings.

2.80 A worried mother brings her 7-year-old daughter who has had a 'menstrual period'.

2.81 An 18-year-old schoolgirl presents with primary amenorrhoea and cyclical lower abdominal pains, and on examination is found to have a blind-ending vagina.

THEME: GENERAL GYNAECOLOGY

A Breast cancer
B Fibroid uterus
C Ovarian tumour
D Pituitary tumour
E Sheehan syndrome
F Turner syndrome
G Vulval tumour

Instructions: From the list above choose the most likely diagnosis associated with the presentations described below. Each option can be used once, more than once or not at all.

2.82 A 67-year-old woman presents with abdominal swelling, a firm hard pelvic mass and ascites.

2.83 A 34-year-old woman presents with secondary amenorrhoea, galactorrhoea and visual fields defects.

2.84 A 30-year-old woman presents with secondary amenorrhoea for 10 months since giving birth. She delivered at home and had major postpartum haemorrhage.

THEME: SUBSTANCE MISUSE IN PREGNANCY

A Acute detoxification programme
B Advise abstinence from all drug use
C Continue pregnancy with no alteration in drug use + allow breast feeding
D Continue pregnancy with no alteration in drug use + prohibit breast feeding
E Methadone substitution programme + allow breast feeding
F Methadone substitution programme + prohibit breast feeding

Instructions: From the list above choose the most appropriate management for the following clinical scenarios. Each option can be used once, more than once or not at all.

2.85 A woman who has been taking only methadone 20 mg/day for 2 years and wishes to continue in her pregnancy. What management plan would you recommend.

2.86 A pregnant woman with an intravenous heroin habit who asks for help to cease heroin use.

2.87 What would you advise a pregnant woman who uses cocaine?

THEME: CONTRACEPTION

A Combined oral contraceptive
B Condoms and combined oral contraceptives
C Depo-Provera injection
D Female sterilisation
E Male sterilisation
F Mirena (levonorgestrel) intrauterine system (IUS)
G Progesterone-only pill

Instructions: From the list above choose the most appropriate contraceptive method for the scenarios given below. Each option can be used once, more than once or not at all.

2.88 A 34-year-old human immunodeficiency virus (HIV)-positive woman, with a partner who is HIV negative, who wishes contraception.

2.89 A 40-year-old single parent with five children who has completed her family.

2.90 A 19-year-old student who has had a termination of pregnancy following an oral contraceptive failure wishes effective contraception. She is about to embark on 6 months travel abroad.

Practice Paper 2
Answers

BEST OF FIVE ANSWERS

2.1 D: Gastroschisis

Gastroschisis is a condition amenable to postnatal treatment and is not lethal.

2.2 B: Request an amniocentesis

Amniocentesis can deliver a rapid result with polymerase chain reaction (PCR) techniques, and it is a safer test than CVS. The woman's age is not relevant as it is analysed as part of the test result. Repeat testing will not clarify the dilemma and a termination is not warranted as the chance of a baby without Down syndrome is 99%.

2.3 D: Phenothiazines are associated with Ebstein anomaly

Phenothiazines are often used for hyperemesis gravidarum and are not associated with congenital malformation. Ebstein anomaly can be caused by lithium.

2.4 D: Following reversal of vasectomy there is an 80% chance of a subsequent pregnancy

Steroids are ineffective in the treatment of antisperm antibodies. Varicocele surgery in not routinely helpful to improve pregnancy rates except with a clinically apparent varicocele in oligozoospermic men.

Questions on pages 75–84

2.5 B: Passage of small pieces of tissue vaginally

Passage of small pieces of tissue vaginally indicate a miscarriage. Multiple sexual partners can lead to pelvic inflammatory disease; adhesions from previous abdominal surgery can also increase the risk of ectopic pregnancy.

2.6 C: The infection can be transmitted to the neonate at the time of delivery

80% of women are asymptomatic. Single dose azithromycin or doxycycline 100 mg twice daily for 14 days are effective treatments. *Chlamydia* can cause neonatal conjunctivitis and pneumonia

2.7 C: Screening should begin at 25 years of age

Screening of teenagers is currently not recommended. First invitation is at 25 years of age, then 3-yearly until 49 years, and then 5-yearly from 50 to 65 years. After 65 years of age only those not screened after 50 years and those with abnormal tests should be screened.

2.8 C: Urge incontinence

Urge, urge incontinence, frequency and nocturia are features of detrusor instability.

2.9 C: Aysymptomatic bacteriuria affects approximately 30% of older women

Females are much more prone to UTIs because of the short urethra. Significant bacteriuria represents a bacterial count of 10^5 CFU/ml. Vaginal oestrogen preparations help in prevention of recurrent UTI in postmenopausal women. Sulphonamides and nitrofurantoin are relatively safe.

2.10 E: 'Stretch and sweep'

Stretch and sweep of the cervix and membranes can be carried out as an outpatient. The safety and effectiveness of the other methods has not been proved.

2.11 C: Visual disturbances

Pedal oedema often exists but is not a criterion for diagnosis of preeclampsia. Features of imminent eclampsia are severe headache, visual disturbances, epigastric pain, hyper-reflexia and clonus.

2.12 B: A woman should not wait for > 3 weeks from the first referral to the time of termination

Legally termination can be performed up to 24 weeks, and later only in exceptional circumstances. A chlamydia screen is routinely offered before termination. Competent girls < 16 years of age can give consent. Suction termination is best performed after 7 weeks of pregnancy. There is a high rate of failure if it is done too early and there is an increased risk of continuation of pregnancy.

2.13 D: Risk of deep vein thrombosis

Laparoscopic sterilisation is usually a day case procedure with not much risk of thrombosis. All the other risks mentioned need to be explained, along with risk of injury to the bowel and bladder, irreversibility of procedure and other available methods of contraception.

2.14 E: Transcutaneous electrical nerve stimulation (TENS) can be sometimes used for relief

TENS may be useful in the relief of chronic pain. Corticosteroids (dexamethasone) can be beneficial for intractable pain and help improve the overall feeling of wellbeing over the short term.

2.15 C: Check her immunity with varicella zoster IgG titre

Varicella infection before 20 weeks of pregnancy causes fetal varicella syndrome in 2% of cases. This is characterised by scarring of skin, eye defects, hypoplasia of the limbs and neurological abnormalities. Eighty-five per cent of women are immune, and therefore can be reassured if their serum varicella zoster IgG is positive.

2.16 A: About 0.3% of women have feto-maternal haemorrhage > 15ml

In some European countries a high dose of anti-D is routinely given to rhesus-negative women without performing a Kleihauer count; however, this policy does not cover 0.3% of women. Up to 50% of large feto-maternal bleeds occur after delivery. Anti-D is not recommended after spontaneous miscarriage before 12 weeks. Prophylactic anti-D is given to non-sensitised women at 28 and 34 weeks.

2.17 C: Intrauterine contraceptive device (IUCD) should be removed in all cases of severe PID

IUCD should not be removed in mild PID, however, it should be removed in severe cases. On the basis of animal studies, ofloxacin should be avoided in young women. Inpatient treatment is needed when a surgical cause is not ruled out; clinically severe disease, tubo-ovarian abscess, and in cases of intolerance to oral treatment. Laparoscopy is not always performed.

2.18 A: Vacuum extraction

The rates of operative delivery have not reduced and are stable at 10–15% in spite of rising lower segment caesarean section rates. The situation described is ideal for a vacuum extraction. Both type of forceps suggested are not used in occipito-transverse positions and a caesarean would be more difficult than a vacuum extraction.

2.19 E: Outlet-instrumental delivery

Outlet instrumental delivery is not associated with increased risk of venous thromboembolism, however, midcavity instrumental delivery and lower segment caesarean section are risk factors for venous thromboembolism. Hyperemesis and dehydration also increase the risk.

2.20 B: Initiating pelvic floor exercises in postpartum period may reduce risk of future urinary incontinence

Moderate aerobic exercise during pregnancy has various benefits, however, exercise in the supine position should be avoided as it can cause vena cava compression by the pregnant uterus. Scuba diving, horse riding, skiing, gymnastics and cycling are also dangerous as they can cause decompression sickness, gas embolism or accidents and fetal trauma.

MULTIPLE CHOICE ANSWERS

2.21 ADE

Klinefelter syndrome characteristically has an XXY chromosome complement. Cri-du-chat syndrome is due to deletion of part of the short arm of chromosome 5. Patau syndrome displays trisomy 13. Tay–Sachs disease is associated with a single autosomal recessive gene and achondroplasia is due to an autosomal dominant gene, neither of which are usually recognisable without using special techniques.

2.22 ABE

There are many forms of medical treatment for endometriosis, but the aim is to induce either a pseudo-pregnancy or a pseudomenopausal state. The progestogens, such as medroxyprogesterone acetate and gestrinone, are helpful. Danazol suppresses the mid-cycle luteinising hormone surge and leads to high androgen gonadotrophin secretion by the pituitary. It has marked androgenic side effects and is rarely used nowadays.

2.23 ABE

An oblique lie is associated with multiparity, uterine abnormality, fundal placenta, pelvic tumours, small pelvic inlet and polyhydramnios. Due to the risk of cord prolapse, admission is recommended at or around 37 weeks' gestation.

2.24 BDE

The incidence of breech presentation is around 20% at 28 weeks with the incidence at term being 3–4%. There is higher perinatal mortality and morbidity with breech presentation principally because of:

- prematurity
- congenital malformation
- birth asphyxia
- birth trauma.

External cephalic version has been subjected to rigorous scientific studies. There is a marked reduction in the risk of Caesarean section in women in whom there is an intention to undertake external cephalic version without any increased risk to the baby.

The Term Breech Trial conducted via the Canadian Medical Research Council was stopped early because it was confirmed that vaginal delivery is more hazardous than elective caesarean section. Perinatal death for term frank/ complete breech fetus with planned caesarean birth was reduced by 75%.

2.25 ACDE

There is an increase in the glomerular filtration rate in normal pregnancy. This leads to an increased excretion of folate and glucose. Because of the latter the renal threshold may be reached and there may be glycosuria. Urate excretion increases by 40%. Ureteric dilatation is known to occur, possibly as a progesterone effect.

2.26 ACDE

The following are all causes of pruritus vulvae:

- Fungal infections
  - *Candida*
  - *Tinea*
- Parasitic infections
  - Scabies
  - Pediculosis pubis
  - Threadworm
- Viral infections
  - Herpes
  - Warts
  - *Molluscum contagiosum*
- Sexually transmitted diseases
  - trichomoniasis
  - gonorrhoea
- Local dermatological conditions
  - Contact dermatitis
  - Psoriasis, etc
- General medical disorders
  - Diabetes mellitus
  - Thyroid disease
  - Liver disease
  - Crohn disease

... *continued*

  - Chronic renal failure
  - Polycythaemia
  - Chronic lymphatic leukaemia
- Vulval dystrophies and tumours
  - Miscellaneous, eg foreign bodies
  - Generalised dermatosis
  - Drug reactions
  - Psychogenic
  - Lichen sclerosus

2.27 AD

Our understanding of the changes in cardiac output in pregnancy has evolved gradually with changes in measurement techniques. The most widely accepted view is that in the normal pregnant woman at rest, not lying supine, cardiac output rises from early pregnancy to peak around 20 weeks' gestation at approximately 5 l/min or 40% above the nonpregnant level; this level seems to be maintained throughout the rest of pregnancy. Although venous pressure in the legs has been shown to increase during pregnancy, that in the arms is unaltered and central venous pressure is said to remain in the range of 2–5 cmH_2O. Peripheral resistance is calculated from the mean arterial pressure divided by cardiac output; as cardiac output is increased and arterial blood pressure if anything falls slightly, it follows that peripheral resistance must be decreased. The fall has been estimated at between 20% and 40% and seems to be maximal in mid-pregnancy; this is due to the opening up of new vascular beds within the uterus and placenta and a general relaxation in peripheral vascular tone. The increased cardiac output of pregnancy is achieved by both an increase in heart rate (averaging 15 bpm) and stroke volume (from 65 ml to 70 ml); again these changes are present from early pregnancy.

2.28 AD

Depo-Provera is the most widely used injectable method of contraception. It is effective, reversible, does not have a deleterious effect on lactation and does not interfere with sexual activity. The failure rate ranges between 0 and 0.7 pregnancies/100 women years. A dose of 150 mg of Depo-Provera effectively suppresses ovulation by inhibiting the secretion of the pituitary gonadotrophins. It alters the yield, composition and physical characteristics of cervical mucus.

2.29 ABCDE

Learn these definitions!

2.30 AE

If looked for at the time of laparoscopy, mild endometriosis is found in about 10% of cases. However, it may be asymptomatic and thus it could be counted as a 'normal' finding. The menopause, either natural or induced, will prevent the recurrence of endometriosis.

2.31 CDE

The following recommendations are based on the Royal College of Obstetricians and Gynaecologists guidelines for rhesus prophylaxis. Anti-D should be given to all non-sensitised rhesus-negative women who:

- miscarry after 12 weeks – whether complete or incomplete
- those who miscarry below 12 weeks when the uterus is evacuated surgically or medically
- threatened miscarriage after 12 weeks
- threatened miscarriage below 12 weeks when the bleeding is heavy or there is abdominal pain.

2.32 ABC

Medical treatment of dysfunctional uterine bleeding depends on the individual woman's medical history as well as her wishes. Progestogens have a limited role if taken orally, but the progestogen-releasing coil is an effective treatment option.

2.33 BC

A cervical smear may be negative in the presence of frank carcinoma. The surface of the malignant tissue is often ulcerated and the sample from the smear shows necrotic debris and possible inflammatory cells. A diagnosis of carcinoma can only be substantiated by cervical biopsy. Inflammatory smears require further investigation to exclude cervical intraepithelial neoplasia (CIN) and human papillomavirus (HPV) infection. Some studies have shown that 10% of inflammatory smears have CIN and > 20% are associated with HPV. *Trichomonas vaginalis* may produce an anti-inflammatory picture that the inexperienced cytologist may find difficult to interpret, but the cells will not be dyskaryotic. Dyskaryotic cells show abnormal nuclear changes: large nuclei with increased chromatin and evidence of mitoses. Koilocytes are cells which appear empty due to the presence of HPV within them. Cervical smears taken at the postnatal clinic at 6 weeks are notoriously inaccurate and are often obscured by inflammatory material from the lochia and necrotic tissue.

2.34 ABCDE

As chicken pox is a highly infectious disease, isolation of patient from other vulnerable pregnant women and neonates is essential. Delivery is ideally delayed for 5–7 days after the onset of the maternal infection to reduce the infection risk to neonate. If, however it cannot be achieved then neonate should be protected by varicella zoster immunoglobin as soon as possible. Pneumonia in pregnant women is severe and has increased mortality therefore treatment with antivirals must be considered.

2.35 D

Sensitive terms that are now preferred are given in the table below.

Older term	New term
Spontaneous abortion	Miscarriage
Incomplete abortion	Incomplete miscarriage
Missed abortion (presence of non-viable fetus)	Silent miscarriage
Anembryonic pregnancy (absent fetal echo)	Delayed miscarriage
	Early fetal demise

Miscarriage occurs in about 10–20% of all clinical pregnancies accounting for about 50 000 inpatient admissions to hospital annually in the UK. This figure may be reducing with the introduction of early pregnancy assessment units (EPAU) and more conservative management. Bedrest does not change the outcome of a threatened miscarriage, rather it may increase the risk of deep vein thrombosis and pulmonary embolism. Medical evacuation and expectant management are accepted optional techniques although they have not replaced surgical evacuation. Several medical methods have been described, including:

- Prostaglandin analogues – gemeprost, misoprostol
- With or without anti-progesterone priming – mifepristone

Serious risks of surgical evacuation are:

- Perforation
- Cervical tears
- Intra-abdominal trauma
- Intrauterine adhesions
- Haemorrhage
- Venous thrombosis and embolism
- Infection

That routine use of antibiotic prophylaxis is reducing the incidence of pelvic infection after induced abortion has been demonstrated. Screening for chlamydia should be offered to all women undergoing surgical treatment of missed miscarriages.

2.36 ADE

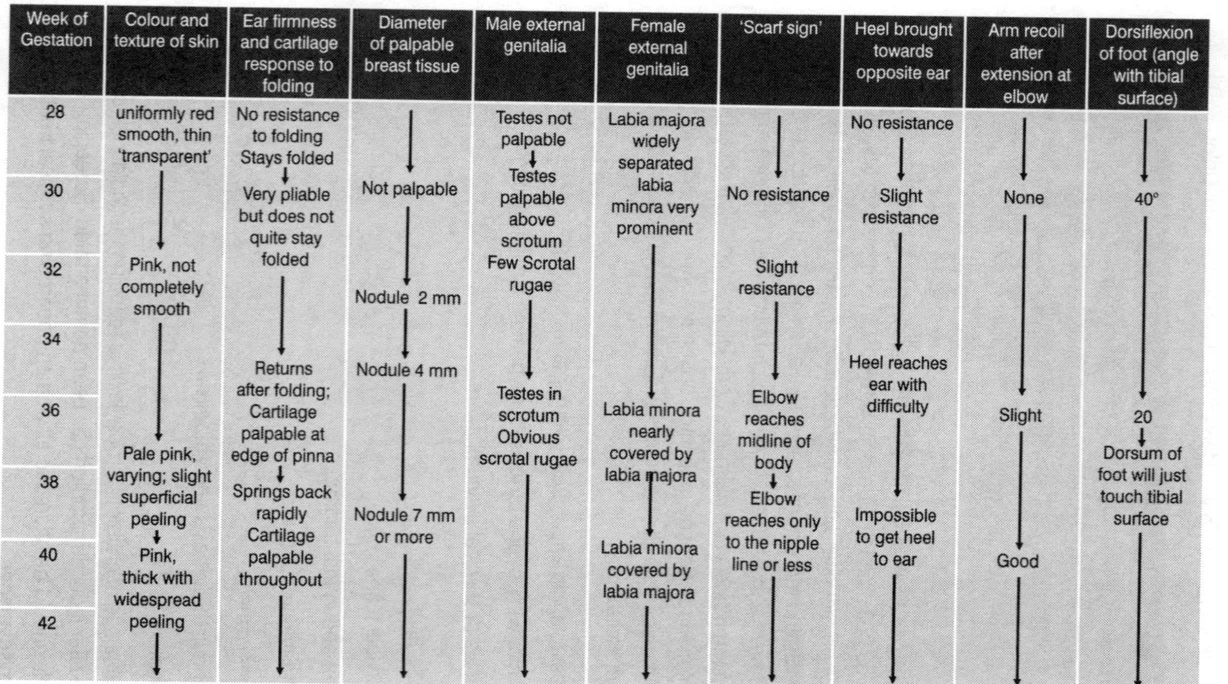

Week of Gestation	Colour and texture of skin	Ear firmness and cartilage response to folding	Diameter of palpable breast tissue	Male external genitalia	Female external genitalia	'Scarf sign'	Heel brought towards opposite ear	Arm recoil after extension at elbow	Dorsiflexion of foot (angle with tibial surface)
28	uniformly red smooth, thin 'transparent'	No resistance to folding Stays folded		Testes not palpable	Labia majora widely separated labia minora very prominent		No resistance		
30		Very pliable but does not quite stay folded	Not palpable	Testes palpable above scrotum Few Scrotal rugae		No resistance	Slight resistance	None	40°
32	Pink, not completely smooth		Nodule 2 mm			Slight resistance			
34			Nodule 4 mm				Heel reaches ear with difficulty		
36		Returns after folding; Cartilage palpable at edge of pinna		Testes in scrotum Obvious scrotal rugae	Labia minora nearly covered by labia majora	Elbow reaches midline of body		Slight	20
38	Pale pink, varying; slight superficial peeling	Springs back rapidly Cartilage palpable throughout	Nodule 7 mm or more			Elbow reaches only to the nipple line or less	Impossible to get heel to ear		Dorsum of foot will just touch tibial surface
40	Pink, thick with widespread peeling				Labia minora covered by labia majora			Good	
42									

2.37 AE

Transvaginal ultrasound is safe and more accurate than transabdominal in locating the placenta. Numerous studies have investigated transvaginal ultrasound for placenta praevia, and none have shown an increase in bleeding. Recent guidelines from the Royal College of Obstetricians and Gynaecologists state that inpatient management is still appropriate for women with major praevia in the third trimester. There is no evidence that cervical cerclage provides any benefit. The mode of delivery should be based on clinical judgement but a placenta encroaching within 2 cm of the internal os is a contraindication to attempting vaginal delivery. Excessive life-threatening bleeding can occur at the time of caesarean section. Techniques to control bleeding include:

- uterotonic agents
- bimanual compression
- aortic compression
- 'B-Lynch' sutures
- internal iliac artery ligation
- hysterectomy.

2.38 ABD

The prevalence of endometriosis in the following conditions is:

- women being investigated for infertility – 20%
- women undergoing sterilisation – 6%
- women being investigated for chronic abdominal pain – 15%
- women undergoing hysterectomy – 25%.

Diagnosis can be based on the following:

- Symptoms (but it may be asymptomatic):
  - Dysmenorrhoea
  - Pelvic pain
  - Infertility
  - Secondary dysmenorrhoea
  - Deep dyspareunia
  - Pelvic pain
- Estimation of gestation of newborn babies
- Signs
  - Abdominal/vaginal tenderness
  - Pelvic mass
- Investigations:
  - Laparoscopy is the gold standard
  - Transvaginal scan – of limited value
  - Magnetic resonance imaging – of limited value
  - CA125 – may be raised and may help to diagnosis or monitor disease progress.

2.39 BDE

Calcium is actively transported across the placenta to the fetus against a concentration gradient. Soon after birth the serum calcium concentration in the baby falls, maximally on the second day. It then rises towards adult values during the next 2–3 days. It is therefore largely unrelated to maternal blood calcium at or around birth and is unlikely to be influenced by maternal dietary deficiency. Hypocalcaemia is seen in babies born to diabetic mothers and in association with neonatal hypoglycaemia. It does not usually cause permanent brain damage, but is a common cause of neonatal tetany and/or convulsions.

2.40 AE

PCOS is a multisystem disorder representing hypothalamic pituitary ovarian/adrenal interaction. Chronic stimulation by luteinising hormone, compounded by hyperinsulinaemia, combined with the overall increased amount of androgen secreting stromal and thecal tissue in the ovary are major reasons for the excessive rate of ovarian androgen secretion in PCOS. Fasting insulin concentrations are raised in 33% of lean and 75% of obese women with PCOS. Insulin and possibly insulin-like growth factor 1 has a gonadotrophic action, promoting ovarian androgen synthesis and thus contributing to menstrual disturbances. Elevated levels of luteinising hormone, leading to a hyperandrogenic environment within the follicle and premature ageing of the oocyte are suggested factors contributing to subfertility and poor pregnancy outcome in patients with PCOS.

2.41 CE

The commonest malignancy causing female deaths is breast cancer. There has not been a marked reduction in total mortality of women with cervical carcinoma in Great Britain. The incidence of the disease is increased in smokers. A Wertheim hysterectomy is the usual treatment in a thin woman, but radiotherapy is used in obese women.

2.42 DE

The table below shows the links mentioned between hormone replacement therapy and different conditions in the recent handbook of the British Menopausal Society (2002) entitled *Management of the Menopause*.

Condition	Hormone replacement therapy
Fibroids	Can cause enlargement but evidence poor
Endometriosis	Small increased risk of disease reactivation, but evidence poor
Cervical cancer and dysplasia	Not contraindicated
Hypertension	Not contraindicated
Valvular heart disease	Not contraindicated
Hyperlipidaemia	Not contraindicated; route depends on lipid profile
Diabetes mellitus	Increased risk of osteoporosis, not contraindicated
Thyroid disease	Increased risk of osteoporosis; not contraindicated
Migraine	Not contraindicated, transdermal route preferred
Epilepsy	Not contraindicated, consider concomitant liver enzyme inducers and osteoporosis risk in phenytoin and carbamazepine users
Parkinson disease	May reduce risk of Parkinson disease, not contraindicated
Gallbladder disease	Increased risk
Liver disease	Transdermal route preferred; liaise with specialist
Crohn/coeliac disease	Increased risk osteoporosis; transdermal route preferred to enhance absorption
Rheumatoid arthritis	Increased risk osteoporosis; no increase in flares
Systemic lupus	Increased risk osteoporosis; no increase in erythematosus flares
Asthma	Small increased risk; no worsening of pre-existing disease
Otosclerosis	No evidence available to contraindicate
Malignant melanoma	No association from epidemiological studies
Post-transplant	Should be considered; increased risk osteoporosis
Renal failure	Should be considered; increased risk early menopause

Table adapted with permission from *Management of the Menopause*, The Handbook of the British Menopause Society, third edition, 2002.

2.43 ABE

Down syndrome involves an excess of chromosome 21 material usually due to trisomy, but in 4%, of cases this does not amount to a separate chromosome. It most often arises due to non-separation of the chromosomes during meiosis. A female with Down syndrome has a 1 in 2 chance of having a normal child. After the age of 40 the risk of an affected child is more than 1 in 100. Although the diagnosis of Down syndrome should be based on cytological culture from placenta or amniotic fluid and genetic studies, it may be associated with reduced serum α-fetoprotein.

2.44 BCDE

The placenta acts as an effective barrier against nearly all bacterial and protozoal invaders (*Toxoplasma* is an exception) and, in general, only viruses can cross it.

2.45 ABD

Prolonged physical contact is required for scabies infestation to occur. The insect moves at a speed of approximately 25 mm/min and, therefore, sexual contact needs to be reasonably prolonged. Symptoms can take up to 2–6 weeks after infestation to appear and the patient complains of itching, particularly worse at night when the body is warm. The diagnosis is made by finding the mite and this is done by scraping the top off the whole length of a burrow with a scalpel, putting the material on a slide with 10% potassium hydroxide solution and looking for the mite under the microscope.

2.46 ABDE

Gestational diabetes is glucose intolerance that appears during pregnancy. Most cases can be treated by dietary measures and there is no convincing evidence that insulin treatment in women with an abnormal glucose tolerance test will actually reduce the perinatal mortality. It does decrease the incidence of fetal macrosomia, but sadly there is no convincing evidence of a decrease in the incidence of operative delivery or birth trauma.

2.47 ABC

LHRH analogues saturate the receptors in the pituitary and therefore prevent recurrence of receptor function. This has been called the medical menopause, but it is a misnomer because the gonadotrophins will be low rather than high as is detected in the menopause. It therefore gives the endocrine picture of hypogonadotrophic hypogonadism, ie eventually low luteinising hormone, low follicle-stimulating hormone and low oestradiol. The patient is likely to complain of menopausal symptoms, including hot flushes, night sweats, dry vagina as well as amenorrhoea. It is useful in the treatment of endometriosis, uterine fibroids and menorrhagia, but it is not of long-term benefit because the side-effects of hypo-oestrogenism, ie osteoporosis, would otherwise occur. Long-term treatment with add-back therapy with tibolone has now been licensed. How long this can be continued remains unclear.

2.48 BC

Oxygenated blood returns from the placenta via the umbilical vein; the umbilical arteries carry deoxygenated blood from fetus to placenta. The ductus venosus provides a direct route of flow for oxygenated blood from the umbilical vein to the inferior vena cava. The foramen ovale connects the atria and is an oblique passage through the interatrial septum, and it closes soon after birth due to the greater left atrial pressure closing the septum primum against the septum secundum. The ductus arteriosus is a wide channel linking the left pulmonary artery with the aorta and joins the aorta distal to the origin of the three branches of the aortic arch.

2.49 C

The baby may appear well immediately after birth; signs usually develop within 1–2 hours. The chest X-ray appearances are suggestive, but not pathognomonic. Antibiotics are not indicated.

2.50 AD

Evidence-based medicine can sometimes bring surprise results. We recommend reading the relevant sections in the BMJ Publishing Group's *Clinical Evidence* (www.clinicalevidence.com), an international resource of the best available evidence for effective healthcare. In the section on hyperemesis *Clinical Evidence* states the following regarding the treatments listed in the question.

Beneficial:	Antihistamines
Likely to be beneficial:	Cyanocobalamin (vitamin B_{12}) Dietary ginger
Unknown effectiveness:	Dietary intervention excluding ginger Acupressure Phenothiazines Pyridoxine (vitamin B_6) Corticosteroids

2.51 CD

Genital warts are benign epidermal growths on the external perianal and perigenital region. They are caused by the human papillomavirus of which there are 70 types with types 6 and 11 usually being the causative factor in immunocompetent people. Without treatment their natural life history is variable: staying the same, increasing in size, or spontaneously resolving. They rarely progress to cancer.

2.52 ABCDE

In vulvodynia most of the women presenting with vulval symptoms will complain of pruritus but a considerable number will complain of vulval pain, burning and rawness. The subsects of vulvodynia are:

- vulvar dermatoses
- cyclic vulvodynia
- vestibular papillomatosis
- vulvar vestibulitis
- essential vulvodynia
- idiopathic vulvodynia.

2.53 AE

The important point to note about this question is the word 'screen'. Ultrasound scanning may be diagnostic for a non-genetic disease, such as spina bifida, but monitoring nuchal fold thickness may be beneficial as a screening test for Down syndrome. Amniocentesis and chorionic villus sampling are both diagnostic tests rather than screening tests for genetic abnormalities. An X-ray would not be a useful screening test. α-Fetoprotein, β-human chorionic gonadotrophin and oestriol are part of the triple test and may help screen for at-risk populations with Down syndrome or other trisomies. α-Fetoprotein and oestriol decrease in these instances, and β-human chorionic gonadotrophin increases. Recent research is directed towards a combination of ultrasound and biochemistry as a screening test.

2.54 AD

The exact incidence of pelvic inflammatory disease is unknown because the disease cannot be diagnosed reliably from clinical symptoms. Laparoscopy allows direct visualisation of the fallopian tubes and is still the best single diagnostic test. It is not used routinely because it is invasive. Pelvic inflammatory disease is the most common gynaecological reason for admission to hospital in the USA but most cases are asymptomatic. Most cases are a result of ascending infection from the cervix. The spread of the infection may be increased by vaginal douching and instrumentation of the cervix.

2.55 E

This question demonstrated the importance of reading the question. It states '... in the third trimester ...'. In the first trimester vaginal scanning is an easier procedure than abdominal scanning, picks up pregnancies at an earlier gestation and does not require the uncomfortable full bladder. Biochemical tests for the assessment of fetal well-being have now fallen out of favour, particularly because of delay in getting the result. On the basis of available studies there appears to be no good evidence that the measurement of human placental lactogen, oestriol, human chorionic gonadotrophin or α-fetoprotein in the third trimester is beneficial in the assessment of fetal well-being. A raised α-fetoprotein level at 16 weeks has a possible association with low birth weight, although the predictive value of this test is low. Less than 30% of the women with an abnormally high level of α-fetoprotein gave birth to a baby with low birth weight or low weight for gestational age. The usefulness of α-fetoprotein screening for conditions other than neural tube defects is poor. With the use of ultrasound scanning, the role of α-fetoprotein as a screening tool has been reduced. Biophysical tests now have a much more important role. These include fetal movement counting, non-stress cardiotocography and fetal biophysical profiling. The role of fetal movement counting alone is controversial. It is known that a reduction or cessation of fetal movements occurs in certain instances before fetal death, but this is by no means 100% predictive. The difficulty is that there are often huge variations in the assessment of fetal kicking. There is also a question of whether, by monitoring the fetal movements, the mother is reassured; this can also have a negative effect in the mother putting some of the blame to herself if an abnormality is detected and not picked up. The non-stress cardiotocogram has been widely used in antenatal care. Doppler blood flow looking at the flow through the umbilical artery and other selective arteries of the baby is now being used as a routine method of assessing the fetus – it is more sensitive than cardiotocographic monitoring.

2.56 CDE

Heart disease is potentially life-threatening in pregnancy. Women with pulmonary vascular disease have a very high risk of dying in pregnancy. Eisenmenger syndrome has a mortality of 30%. Careful counselling must be given with the acceptance that there may be a cultural pressure to have a child. It is important to recognise that women may minimise or even deny cardiac symptoms. Endocarditis should always be on your list of differential diagnosis in women with an obscure febrile illness. Oxytocin must be used with caution with the risk of blood pressure changes and tachycardia. If oxytocin is required it should be given by a slow infusion and a maximum daily dose of 5 IU should not be exceeded.

2.57 ABCDE

It was noted in the early 1970s that the rate of death was much higher among infants in the developing world who were fed formula than among infants who were breast fed. This was because of malnutrition and recurrent infectious diseases. Breast feeding was associated with decreased death rates due to acute respiratory infections and diarrhoea in infants aged 1–11 months in Bangladesh when compared with infants who were partially breast fed. Breast feeding has also been found to be protective against enterotoxigenic *Escherichia coli* in the first year of life and to be associated with decreased incidence of *Giardia* infection. The many anti-infective factors found in breast milk include: immunoglobulins (IgA, IgM, IgG), lactoferrin, *Lactobacillus bifidus* growth factor, T and B cell lymphocytes, plasma cells and neutrophils.

Many studies have shown that exclusive breast feeding for 4 months delays the first episode of otitis media and decreased recurrent otitis media. British studies have shown that breast-fed infants had fewer hospital admissions with bronchiolitis than non-breast-fed infants.

2.58 ABCDE

Oblique and transverse lies occur due to the fetus failing to adopt a longitudinal lie. This is associated with:

- the abdominal laxity of multiparity
- congenital fetal abnormalities, especially those that cause polyhydramnios
- uterine abnormalities, especially mild uterine abnormalities, such as subseptate uterus
- shortening of the longitudinal axis of the uterus by fundal or low-lying placenta
- conditions that prevent the engagement of the presenting part, including pelvic tumours and a small pelvic inlet.

2.59 ABDE

Growth restriction in later gestation and a low weight gain in infancy may be associated with an early menopause. It is interesting that the menopause occurs earlier in smokers and smoking causes a reduction in oestrogen. Remember the menopause is one day in a women's life, ie her last period. The climacteric is at the time when a women changes from being able to being unable to sexually reproduce.

2.60 ABCDE

OHSS is a complication of induction of ovulation. It usually occurs after human chorionic gonadotrophin (hCG) has been given and also with luteal phase support with hCG. Women of a younger age, women with polycystic ovarian syndrome and those who have a history of OHSS are at a higher risk. Early pregnancy which produces endogenous hCG is also a predisposing factor. Mild ovarian hyperstimulation presents with abdominal discomfort, swelling and pain and treatment is conservative. Moderate ovarian hyperstimulation often presents with nausea, vomiting and diarrhoea as well as weight gain. Severe hyperstimulation, which is rare, is more serious and pericardial and pleural effusions may develop. Close observation is important and very careful fluid balance and electrolyte monitoring is essential. Fatalities are recognised, due not only to pulmonary embolism but also to renal failure.

EXTENDED MATCHING QUESTIONS ANSWERS

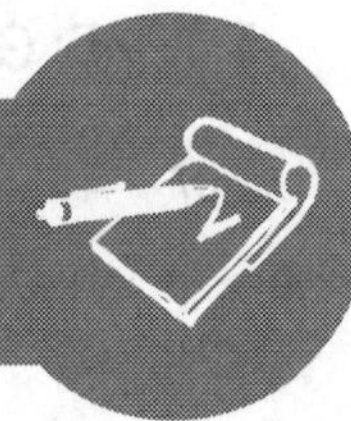

THEME: PRE-PREGNANCY COUNSELLING – RECURRENCE RISKS

2.61 C 10–15%

2.62 C 10–15%

2.63 C 10–15%

THEME: EARLY PREGNANCY PROBLEMS

2.64 H Serum hCG estimation. A event related to pregnancy needs to be diagnosed (or excluded) before further management is planned.

2.65 B Evacuation of uterus. An incomplete miscarriage has been diagnosed.

2.66 G Repeat ultrasound of the uterus in 1 week. Two ultrasound scans 1 week apart is necessary to confirm a failed pregnancy before 8 weeks' gestation.

Questions on pages 101–110

THEME: GENERAL GYNAECOLOGY

2.67 A A 6-month course of GnRH analogues would shrink the fibroids during this window period and has reversible effects that would allow the return of fertility.

2.68 E An endometrial sample should be taken in women above the age of 45 with considerable abnormal uterine bleeding.

2.69 C The combined oral contraceptive is ideal as it would reduce menstrual flow.

THEME: HORMONE REPLACEMENT THERAPY

2.70 G Stop HRT. HRT that is oestrogen-based is associated with an increased risk of breast cancer and is contraindicated in those with a history of breast cancer.

2.71 E HRT is contraindicated in those with a strong family history of deep vein thrombosis and breast cancer in first-degree relatives.

2.72 F HRT is indicated as it controls vasomotor symptoms and prevents osteoporosis.

THEME: INTRA-UTERINE GROWTH RESTRICTION

2.73 C Induction of labour at term. If the umbilical artery Doppler examination is normal there is no urgency. If growth is on the 10th centile it is probably a normal but small fetus.

2.74 A Caesarean section. Absent flow in the umbilical artery indicates fetal hypoxia/acidosis therefore a caesarean is indicated rather than an induction of labour.

2.75 F Ultrasound for fetal growth. This is a low-risk situation and confirmation of the small size of the fetus is necessary before management is planned. The fetus may be normal on ultrasound.

THEME: VACCINATION IN PREGNANCY

2.76 A There is a high risk of developing the disease. A hepatitis B vaccination programme should be commenced.

2.77 E Unsafe, do not give in pregnancy. The woman should be vaccinated after delivery to protect her in any future pregnancy.

2.78 A Hepatitis A vaccination should be given if indicated.

THEME: MENSTRUAL DISORDERS

2.79 D Premature ovarian failure. There may be a history of siblings having had similar presentation as it can run in families.

2.80 C Precocious puberty. Menses beginning before the age of 10 years are abnormal and need to be investigated further to find the cause.

2.81 B Haematocolpos. The history is a classic presentation.

THEME: GENERAL GYNAECOLOGY

2.82 C Ovarian tumour is the most likely cause in a 67-year-old especially as there is a hard mass associated with ascites.

2.83 D Pituitary tumour is likely due to the presence of galactorrhoea in association with visual field defects. The tumour is interfering with the pituitary–ovarian axis causing amenorrhoea.

2.84 E Sheehan syndrome. This syndrome of pituitary failure develops after delivery where there has been considerable postpartum haemorrhage that interferes with the blood supply to the pituitary gland.

THEME: SUBSTANCE MISUSE IN PREGNANCY

2.85 C Continue pregnancy with no alteration in drug use + allow breast feeding. Continuation of the current programme is recommend as problems are not common on such a low dose of methadone. Withdrawal of methadone needs a motivated patient to succeed. Breast feeding is allowed with methadone use as a small amount of methadone is secreted in the breast milk which may help neonatal withdrawal symptoms.

2.86 E Methadone substitution programme + allow breast feeding. A methadone substitution programme is a well described management strategy. Neonatal abstinence is usual in babies when delivered in women who consume large amounts of opiates. Breast feeding could reduce the severity of the abstinence symptoms.

2.87 B Advise abstinence from all drug use. There is no substitution therapy for cocaine withdrawal and psychological addiction is a problem.

THEME: CONTRACEPTION

2.88 B Condoms will protect the partner from HIV infection and allow the couple to have a sexual relationship. Additional contraception is advisable in case of condom failure.

2.89 D Female sterilisation. This is a permanent method of contraception and is suitable for someone who has completed her family.

2.90 F Mirena IUS. This form of contraception is suitable for someone who may not remember to take a pill every day.

Practice Paper 3 Questions

BEST OF FIVE QUESTIONS

20 Questions: Time allowed 30 minutes. Please give the single most appropriate answer from the list of alternatives.

3.1 You are requested to perform a ventouse delivery by a midwife on labour ward. In which one of the following situations is it possible to conduct a ventouse delivery?

- A Face presentation
- B Vertex deflexed at +1 station
- C Breech presentation for delivery of the after coming head
- D Preterm delivery < 34 weeks of pregnancy
- E Maternal hepatitis B infection

3.2 You are asked to perform a forceps delivery for a cephalic presentation. Which one of the following is not a prerequisite to conduct a forceps delivery?

- A Fully dilated cervix
- B Direct occipito-anterior position
- C Ruptured membranes
- D Adequate analgesia
- E Head below ischial spines (o-station)

Answers on pages 187–191

3.3 You see a 24-year-old woman in your clinic who has been having lower abdominal pain on and off for the past 6 months. She has been admitted to different wards on different occasions. Which one of the following is the most appropriate statement regarding her management?

- A Could have been treated as chronic pelvic pain if duration of symptoms was more than 12 months
- B Addressing psychological and social issues may be important in resolving symptoms
- C Symptom-based diagnostic criteria cannot be used with confidence to make the diagnosis of irritable bowel syndrome
- D Diagnostic laparoscopy should be the first line of investigation
- E Ovarian suppression with gonadotrophin releasing hormone

3.4 With regard to induction of labour, which one of the following statements is correct?

- A During induction of labour with prostaglandin fetal heart monitoring is unnecessary
- B Induction of labour with prostaglandin in a woman with a previous caesarean section does not increase the risk of scar dehiscence
- C Ultrasound in the first trimester reduces the induction rates for post-term pregnancy
- D Women with uncomplicated pregnancy should be offered induction after 40 weeks
- E Sweeping and stretching should be offered to all women at 38 weeks' gestation

3.5 A 35-year-old para 3 wishes to have tubal sterilisation. Which one of the following statements is most appropriate?

- A Laparoscopic tubal occlusion should only be performed in a hospital with facilities to perform a laparotomy
- B Laparoscopic sterilisation should be discouraged as it is associated with irregular and heavy periods
- C Diathermy use for sterilisation would be the best option
- D Sterilisation should not be performed as a day case
- E Vasectomy is a more difficult procedure and carries high failure risk compared with tubal sterilisation, therefore it is not advisable

3.6 A 38-year-old woman has been found to have 5 cm anterior wall intramural and 2 cm submucosal fibroid. What is her one most likely presentation?

- A Pressure symptoms involving urinary and bowel functions
- B Sarcomatous changes
- C Polycythemia is due to secretion of an erythropoietin-like substance
- D Infertility
- E Heavy painful periods

3.7 A 35-year-old 6 week' pregnant nurse is keen to have biochemical screening for Down syndrome. Which one maternal serum hormonal level measurement is useful as part of a screening programme?

A α-Fetoprotein

B Human placental lactogen

C Oestradiol

D Prolactin

E Progesterone

3.8 A para 1 with a previous lower segment caesarean section (LSCS) has an anterior placenta praevia in this pregnancy. You are doing her preoperative assessment and taking consent. Which one of the following risks is most important to mention in this specific case while consenting the patient for LSCS?

A Risk of deep vein thrombosis

B Risk of wound infection

C Possible need for hysterectomy

D Risk of future infertility

E Baby's admission to the neonatal unit

3.9 A 30-year-old women with history of deep vein thrombosis wants to use progesterone-only pills for contraception. Which one of the following conditions you will like to rule out before you prescribe her these pills?

- A History of endometriosis
- B Bottle feeding a baby
- C Active liver disease
- D Peptic ulcer
- E Lactation

3.10 A 50-year-old menopausal woman had a cervical smear. The result is reported as inadequate. Her previous smears have been normal. Examination revealed an atrophic vagina and cervix. Which one of the following is the most appropriate management plan for her?

- A Reassure and discharge
- B Refer to colposcopy clinic
- C Do another smear using liquid-based cytology
- D
- E Repeat smear in 6 months' time

3.11 A couple has been trying to conceive for 3 years. Semen analysis results suggest oligozoospermia. Which one factor in the history of the male partner could contribute to his problems?

A Cimetidine medication

B Hypothermia

C Metronidazole medication

D Nitrofurantoin medication

E Tetracycline medication

3.12 With regard to management of twin pregnancy which one of the following practices is an acceptable part of clinical practice?

A Weekly scans to monitor growth and liquor

B Patient should be assessed for premature cervical dilatation by digital examination

C Hospital-based delivery with facilities for electronic fetal monitoring

D Induction of labour/lower segment caesarean section at 37 weeks for all twins

E Physiological management of the third stage of labour

3.13 A gravida 3 para 2 has haemoglobin 9.5 gm/l. She also has pre-eclampsia and gestational diabetes, and presents at 32 weeks with a clinically small baby. Ultrasound confirms asymmetric intra-uterine growth restriction (IUGR) and reduced umbilical artery Doppler flow. She wants to know the possible cause for IUGR. Which one of the following is the most likely cause of IUGR in this case?

- A Intrauterine infections
- B Chromosomal abnormalities
- C Anaemia
- D Pre-eclampsia
- E Gestational diabetes

3.14 You are attending to an 18-year-old university student after a night out. She is requesting emergency contraception. She is taking a contraceptive pill, but she often forgets to take it. Which one of the following is the most important investigation you would like to perform before you prescribe her emergency contraception?

- A High vaginal swab
- B Urine pregnancy test
- C Venereal disease research laboratory (VDRL) estimation
- D Human immunodeficiency virus (HIV) check
- E *Chlamydia* screening

3.15 Which one of the following maternal cardiac diseases is least likely to cause complications during pregnancy?

- A Marfan syndrome
- B Cardiomyopathy
- C Ventricular septal defect
- D Mitral stenosis
- E Pulmonary hypertension

3.16 A diabetic woman on insulin has just delivered, and the baby has been admitted to the neonatal unit. Which one of the following conditions is most likely to be the reason for the neonatal admission in this case?

- A Poor muscle tone
- B Hypoglycaemia
- C Hypothermia
- D Hypercalcaemia
- E Convulsions

3.17 A 44-year-old generally healthy woman presents with symptoms of sensory urgency since a month. There is no haematuria. Considering the differential diagnosis which one of the following is the most likely cause for her symptoms?

A Idiopathic

B Bladder stone

C Carcinoma of bladder

D Cystocele

E Pelvic mass

3.18 A 40-year-old woman presents with symptoms of regular heavy periods. Transvaginal scan shows an intramyometrial fibroid, 6 cm in size. You are discussing various options with her, and she is anxious and wants to avoid surgery. Which one of the following treatments is the best option for her?

A Iron and folate supplements

B Dilatation and curettage

C Intrauterine contraceptive device (IUCD)

D Mirena (levonorgestrel) coil

E Progesterone

3.19 A postmenopausal 55-year-old woman is recently diagnosed with lichen sclerosus on vulval biopsy. You are discussing with her this report and the condition. Which one of the following is not appropriate to mention?

- A It can also involve trunk and limbs in some patients
- B It has an autoimmune aetiology
- C Vulval carcinoma can occur in about 30% of cases
- D Management may require bland emollient cream and steroids
- E Need for follow up

3.20 A 38-year-old smoker with a body mass index (BMI) of 20 kg/m^2 presents with secondary amenorrhoea since a year. Her follicle-stimulating hormone (FSH) level is 50. She is newly married and trying to conceive. Which one of the following is the best possible management available to help her conceive?

- A Induction of ovulation by clomifene
- B Induction of ovulation with gonadotrophins
- C Hormone replacement therapy (HRT)
- D Egg donation and in vitro fertilisation (IVF)
- E Intrauterine insemination

MULTIPLE CHOICE QUESTIONS

40 Questions: Time allowed 1½ hours. Indicate your answers clearly by putting a tick against the correct or true options and a cross against the incorrect or false options. (The section on answers in this book lists the correct (true) options.)

3.21 Maternal mortality is markedly increased in the presence of:

- A Marfan syndrome
- B Valvular heart disease treated by curative surgery
- C Inoperable cyanotic congenital heart disease
- D Primary pulmonary hypertension
- E Congestive cardiomyopathy

3.22 Causes of precocious puberty include:

- A Central neurological lesions
- B Polycystic ovarian syndrome
- C Chronic hyperthyroidism
- D Polycystic kidneys
- E McCune–Albright syndrome

Answers on pages 193–210

3.23 Congenital varicella syndrome:

- A Is secondary to primary varicella zoster infections
- B Is associated with Down syndrome
- C Is associated with skin scarring
- D Is associated with learning disabilities
- E Occurs after 20 weeks' gestation

3.24 Ovulation

- A Is best assessed using basal body temperature
- B Is associated with a mid-luteal rise in progesterone
- C Can be demonstrated on an ultrasound scan
- D Can be detected by a rise in luteinising hormone
- E Is followed by a withdrawal bleed after 12–16 days if pregnancy does not occur

3.25 Pre-eclampsia:

- A Most commonly occurs in women in their first pregnancy
- B Is best treated with antihypertensive treatment and bedrest
- C Is negatively associated with smoking
- D Has an increased incidence in diabetic pregnancies
- E The primary pathology is in the kidneys

3.26 Sex-linked genetic conditions include:

A The hairy pinna trait

B Cleft palate

C Hurler syndrome (type I mucopolysaccharidosis)

D Achondroplasia

E Congenital ichthyosis

3.27 With regard to uterine fibroids:

A They need to be removed surgically in women with secondary infertility

B The incidence of sarcomatous change is 1–2%

C The symptoms can be effectively treated medically

D They are more likely to occur after prolonged use of an oral contraceptive

E They are associated with heavy periods in more than 50% of cases

3.28 With regard to bone and the menopause:

A Osteoporosis is a systematic skeletal disease characterised by micro-architectural deterioration of bony tissues with resultant decreased fragility

B Approximately 15% of women aged above 50 have osteoporosis

C Osteopenia is defined as bone mineral density less than –1.0 SD below the young adult mean to less than –2.5 SD

D Osteoporosis is defined as a bone mineral density of ≥ –2.5 SD below the young adult mean

E The T score is a value that is defined based on a mean axial bone mineral density relative to young healthy adult women

3.29 Recognised causes of recurrent spontaneous miscarriage include:

A Polycystic ovarian syndrome

B Maternal diabetes

C Maternal *Brucella* infection

D Chromosomal abnormalities of the fetus

E Intercourse

3.30 Drugs that cross the placental barrier include:

A Heparin

B Tetracycline

C Sulphadimidine

D Diazepam

E Salicylate

3.31 Cervical eversion:

A Is often found in postmenopausal women

B Should always be investigated by cervical smear

C Can cause chronic vaginal discharge

D If asymptomatic, should still be treated

E Can be treated with coagulation of the cervix

3.32 With regard to management of genital herpes in pregnancy:

A Concern is raised because of neonatal herpes

B If a woman presents with the first attack of genital herpes, she should be referred to a genitourinary physician

C Treatment with aciclovir should be considered for women with first attack

D Caesarean section is the mode of choice for all women who present with first attack of genital herpes in the first trimester

E For women presenting with recurrent genital herpes lesion, the risk to the baby is small

3.33 The vaginal contraceptive diaphragm:

A Is graded in 15 mm sizes

B Should be removed within 2 hours of intercourse

C Is recommended in case of prolapse

D Should be checked if the patient's weight changes by more than 3 kg (7 lb)

E Should be replaced annually

3.34 With regard to eclampsia:

- A Incidence in UK is 4.9/10 000 maternities
- B 44% of eclampsias occur postnatally
- C 38% of eclampsias occur antepartum
- D Maternal fatality rate is 1.8%
- E 35% of women will have one major complication

3.35 The baby of a diabetic mother has:

- A A greater risk of congenital heart disease than a baby of a non-diabetic mother
- B A five-fold increase in risk of respiratory distress syndrome
- C A 10% risk of developing diabetes
- D A greatly increased risk of learning disabilities
- E A risk of hypomagnesaemia in the neonatal period

3.36 Evidence-based treatment options for endometriosis causing pain include:

- A Non-steroidal drugs
- B Combined oral contraceptive
- C Gonadotrophin releasing hormone agonist
- D Laparoscopic ablation
- E Continuous progestogens

3.37 The fetal head:

- A May be at the ischial spines but not engaged
- B Can be delivered vaginally in a mento-posterior position
- C Will display the Spalding sign within 24 hours of intrauterine death
- D May undergo asynclitism in negotiating the pelvic outlet
- E Is likely to be a vertex presentation when deflexed

3.38 With regard to human chorionic gonadotrophin:

- A It is produced by the trophoblast
- B It is produced by the fetal liver
- C It may be immunosuppressive
- D The serum level peaks in the second trimester of pregnancy
- E It is produced by some non-trophoblastic tumours

3.39 In the menstrual cycle:

- A Ovulation follows the luteinising hormone surge by 48 hours
- B Oestradiol stimulates endometrial cell proliferation in the proliferative phase
- C Progesterone, in the secretory phase, produces vacuolation of the cell with the nuclei displaced towards the gland lumen
- D Bleeding is caused by failure of implantation and a cessation of oestrogen production
- E Early production of trophoblastic human chorionic gonadotrophin maintains the corpus luteum and thus prevents the withdrawal bleed

3.40 Endometrial carcinoma:

A Frequently occurs in women aged 30–34

B Is associated with unopposed progestogens

C Is treated by radiotherapy

D Can be diagnosed by ultrasound scanning

E Has a poor prognosis

3.41 With regard to Apgar scores:

A Heart rate: > 100 bpm = 2

B Colour: blue and pale = 0

C Muscle tone: some limb flexion = 1

D Respiratory effort: slow and irregular = 1

E Eye movement: irregular = 0

3.42 With regard to ectopic pregnancy:

A Rarely it is associated with in vitro fertilisation

B Diagnosis can be excluded by ultrasound scanning

C Surgery is the only treatment

D It is associated with maternal death

E It can be excluded if a gestational sac is seen within the uterus

3.43 Serum α-fetoprotein is likely to be raised in:

- A Spina bifida occulta
- B Down syndrome
- C Threatened abortion
- D Exomphalos
- E Multiple pregnancy

3.44 With regard to bacterial vaginosis:

- A It is less common than *Candida* infection
- B It is caused by the lactobacilli
- C The vaginal pH is greater than 4.5
- D It is associated with a fishy odour
- E It may be associated with preterm labour

3.45 The typical female bony pelvis:

- A Has a transverse diameter at the inlet greater than the anteroposterior diameter
- B Has an obstetric conjugate of 11–12 cm
- C Is funnel-shaped
- D Has an obtuse greater sciatic notch
- E Has a subpubic angle greater than 90°

3.46 Fetal pulmonary maturity:

A Is delayed in diabetic pregnancies

B Normally occurs before the 36th week of gestation

C Is influenced by corticosteroid levels

D Is controlled by α-fetoprotein

E Is always delayed in cases of learning disabilities

3.47 Tumours that arise in the ovary are:

A Nephroblastoma

B Cystadenoma

C Granulosa cell tumour

D Neuroblastoma

E Teratoma

3.48 Amniocentesis in the second trimester:

A Is associated with an overall pregnancy loss more than 3% that of matched controls

B Carries a greater risk of fetal wastage when the placenta is implanted anteriorly as opposed to posteriorly

C Is indicated in a woman whose female cousin has previously delivered a child with a neural tube defect

D Carries a diagnostic error rate of around 10% in chromosomal analysis

E Is associated with a 2% risk of failure of the cells to culture

3.49 ***Chlamydia trachomatis*****:**

A Has an intracellular existence

B Causes psittacosis

C Is associated with Fitz–Hugh–Curtis syndrome

D Is best treated by penicillin derivatives

E Can only be detected by the measurement of a heat-stable antigen

3.50 With regard to postpartum haemorrhage (PPH):

A The most frequent cause is uterine atony

B Risk factors include previous PPH

C Primary PPH occurs within 72 hours after delivery

D Secondary PPH occurs in approximately 10% of all deliveries

E Intramuscular or intramyometrial prostaglandin (Hemabate; 0.25 mg) can be used for uterine atony

3.51 Nausea and vomiting:

A Are among the most troublesome symptoms of early pregnancy

B In early pregnancy are usually due to a rise in oestrogen levels

C Can be treated with antihistamines which are considered to be safe in pregnancy

D In late pregnancy can be associated with preeclampsia

E Can be the presenting feature of a hydatidiform mole

3.52 Premature ovarian failure may be due to:

A Chromosome abnormalities

B Autoimmune disease

C Metabolic disease

D Chemotherapy

E Hysterectomy and conservation of ovaries

3.53 In the days following ovulation:

A The basal body temperature falls

B The endometrium undergoes secretory changes

C The plasma progesterone concentration falls

D Cervical mucus becomes scanty and more viscous

E Plasma luteinising hormone level falls

3.54 With regard to antepartum haemorrhage:

A It may be due to a cervical eversion

B It may be treated with rest at home if the cervix is closed

C Rhesus-negative patients should be given anti-D immunoglobulin

D It is associated with an increased incidence of postpartum haemorrhage

E If due to placental abruption, blood loss is a good indicator of severity

3.55 Which of following should be discussed with a woman before agreeing to carry out a sterilisation:

A There is a failure rate of approximately 10%

B Is she aware that reversal is possible

C It is routinely performed by laparoscopic electrodiathermy of the tubes

D It will make her periods heavier

E Has her partner considered a vasectomy

3.56 Increasing maternal age is associated with:

A Increased risk of Down syndrome

B Decreased risk of miscarriage

C Decreased risk of monozygotic twins

D Increased risk of hydatidiform moles

E Decreased risk of postpartum haemorrhage

3.57 Genital herpes:

A Is usually caused by the organism which causes lip herpes

B Is often recurrent

C Is usually transmitted sexually

D If uncomplicated will heal without treatment in about 10 days

E Should be treated with penicillin if secondary infection develops

3.58 With regard to perimenopausal contraception:

A Female sterilisation is the most commonly used method of contraception in the age group of 40–49 years

B Women should stop taking the combined oral contraceptive at the age of 45

C Progestogen-only pill should only be used in women for whom the combined oral contraceptive is contraindicated

D A copper-containing intrauterine device inserted after the age of 40 can be left until contraception is no longer required

E Emergency combined hormonal contraception can be used in this group

3.59 Which of the following definitions is/are correct?

A Secondary amenorrhoea – the absence of menses for 6 months in a previously menstruating woman

B Dysfunctional uterine bleeding – excessive or prolonged regular menstrual bleeding in the absence of overt uterine, endocrine or haematological disorder

C Climacteric – the last menstrual period

D Puberty – the first menstrual period

E Dysmenorrhoea – painful vaginal bleeding

3.60. In *'Why Mothers Die 2000-2002'*:

- A Thrombosis and thromboembolism remain the major indirect causes of maternal death
- B Thrombosis and thromboembolism account for 25-30% of all direct maternal deaths
- C Hypertensive disease of pregnancy remains the third leading cause of direct deaths
- D Haemorrhage is the 5th leading cause of direct deaths.
- E Deaths in early pregnancy are mostly related to legal terminations of pregnancy

EXTENDED MATCHING QUESTIONS

30 Questions: Time allowed 1 hour.

THEME: GENETICS

A 1 in 2 chance
B 1 in 2 chance of males affected
C 1 in 2 chance of females affected
D 1 in 4 chance
E 1 in 8 chance
F No pattern of inheritance
G Not genetic

Instructions: From the list above choose the most appropriate description of risk that matches the diseases given below. Each option can be used once, more than once or not at all.

3.61 A couple with a child with cystic fibrosis ask about their chance of an affected child in a future pregnancy.

3.62 A woman with a son with haemophilia asks about the chance of another child having the disease.

3.63 A man who has Duchenne muscular dystrophy would like to know the chance of his son being affected.

Answers on pages 211–214

THEME: PRENATAL DIAGNOSIS

A 1%
B 2%
C 5%
D 15–25%
E 30–40%
F 60–70%
G > 90%

Instructions: From the list above choose the correct estimation for each of the following questions related to screening and diagnostic tests. Each option can be used once, more than once or not at all.

3.64 The approximate detection rate for a fetus with Down syndrome when second trimester biochemical screening is used (eg the triple test), with maternal age for a false positive rate of 5%.

3.65 The approximate detection rate for a fetus with Down syndrome when nuchal translucency is combined with serum biochemical screening (associated plasma protein (PAPP-A), β-human chorionic gonadotrophin (hCG)) and maternal age for a false positive rate of 5%.

3.66 The approximate detection rate for a fetus with Down syndrome when maternal age alone is used as a screening test (false positive rate of 5%).

THEME: MISCARRIAGE

A Complete miscarriage
B Incomplete miscarriage
C Inevitable miscarriage
D Missed miscarriage
E Recurrent miscarriages
F Threatened miscarriage

Instructions: From the list above choose the most appropriate diagnosis for women in early pregnancy presenting your general practice. Each option can be used once, more than once or not at all.

3.67 A booking ultrasound scan reveals a gestational sac of 22 mm with no fetal pole.

3.68 The woman presents with bleeding, positive pregnancy test, a fetal heart beat seen on ultrasound and closed cervical os.

3.69 On vaginal examination, some products of conception are seen in the cervical canal and the cervical os is open.

THEME: CONTRACEPTION

A Combined oral contraceptives
B Copper intrauterine contraceptive device
C Implanon
D Depo-Provera
E Levonelle and condoms
F Low-dose progesterone pills
G Mirena (levonorgestrel) intrauterine system (IUS)
H Spermicides

Instructions: From the list above choose the most appropriate contraceptive advice that you will give to the following females presenting to your practice. Each option can be used once, more than once or not at all.

3.70 A 17-year-old schoolgirl has had unprotected sexual intercourse 4 hours ago and is requesting emergency contraception.

3.71 A 15-year-old schoolgirl who is going for surgical termination of pregnancy.

3.72 A 40-year-old mother of three who is a heavy smoker and has heavy periods requests contraception.

THEME: GYNAECOLOGICAL CANCER

A BRCA gene mutations
B Combined oral contraceptives
C Human papilloma virus
D Mirena (levonorgestrel) intrauterine system (IUS)
E Neisseria gonorrhoea
F Tamoxifen
G Vulval warts

Instructions: From the list of above of factors that may be causative or associated with gynaecological malignancies choose the factors appropriate for the malignancies given below. Each option can be used once, more than once or not at all.

3.73 Endometrial cancer

3.74 Cervical cancer

3.75 Ovarian cancer

THEME: ABDOMINAL PAIN IN PREGNANCY

A Abortion/miscarriage
B Appendicitis
C Cholecystitis
D Fibroids
E Placental abruption
F Preterm labour
G Round ligament tendinitis
H Torsion of ovarian cyst

Instructions: From the list above choose the most likely diagnosis for the scenarios described below. Each option can be used once, more than once or not at all.

3.76 A woman at 32 weeks' gestation with constant central abdominal pain, no vomiting/diarrhoea. Kleihauer test is positive.

3.77 A woman with a 2-day history of vomiting and no diarrhoea at 36 weeks' gestation. She complains of constant central abdominal pain. There is a mild pyrexia and slight tenderness and guarding in the right flank.

3.78 A woman at 26 weeks' gestation with lower abdominal pain and mild vomiting. There is a low-grade pyrexia and tenderness over the uterus bilaterally.

THEME: PRETERM RUPTURE OF MEMBRANES

A Atosiban infusion
B Augment labour with oxytocin
C Caesarean section
D Co-amoxiclav orally
E Conservative management with no medication
F Corticosteroids
G Erythromycin orally
H Nifedipine orally

Instructions: From the list above choose the most appropriate management for the scenarios described below. In each scenario the fetus is thought to be healthy with no growth restriction or fetal abnormalities. Each option can be used once, more than once or not at all.

3.79 Ruptured membranes, no contractions, at 24 weeks' gestation.

3.80 Ruptured membranes for 2 weeks' duration, now at 30 weeks' gestation with the onset of contractions. Cephalic presentation.

3.81 Ruptured membranes, no contractions, with a footling breech presentation at 28 weeks' gestation.

THEME: ANAESTHESIA IN OBSTETRICS

A Epidural anaesthesia
B General anaesthetic
C Immersion in warm water
D Non-steroidal drugs
E Pethidine (intramuscular)
F Spinal anaesthesia
G Transcutaneous nerve stimulation (TENS)

Instructions: From the list above choose the most appropriate method of analgesia in the following circumstances. The fetus is healthy unless otherwise stated. Each option can be used once, more than once or not at all.

3.82 Pain relief in labour for a woman with an intrauterine death following placental abruption.

3.83 Pain relief in labour in a woman who is taking methadone 40 mg/day as part of a maintenance programme.

3.84 Emergency caesarean section for cephalopelvic disproportion (no analgesia has been given previously).

THEME: GENERAL GYNAECOLOGY

A Chronic pelvic inflammatory disease
B Endometriosis
C Ovarian cysts
D Pelvic adhesions
E Pelvic congestion
F Psychogenic pain
G Uterine displacement

Instructions: Chronic pelvic pain can have various underlying pathologies. From the list above choose the condition which best describes the clinical situations below. Each option can be used once, more than once or not at all.

3.85 A 31-year-old woman with chronic pelvic pain associated with dyspareunia and dysmenorrhoea.

3.86 A 25-year-old woman with a history of subfertility, vaginal discharge and chronic pelvic pain.

3.87 A 33-year-old woman with a history of multiple abdominal surgery and chronic pelvic pain.

THEME: GENERAL GYNAECOLOGY

A Eisenmenger syndrome
B Meigs syndrome
C Ovarian hyperstimulation syndrome
D Polycystic ovary syndrome
E Premenstrual syndrome
F Turner syndrome

Instructions: From the list above choose the clinical syndrome which best fits women presenting with the following signs and symptoms. Each option can be used once, more than once or not at all.

3.88 A 21-year-old woman presents with a webbed neck and primary amenorrhoea.

3.89 A 42-year-old woman is found to have a triad of ascites, right-sided pleural effusion and an ovarian fibroma.

3.90 A couple attends an infertility clinic and the woman is found to have oligomenorrhoea.

Practice Paper 3 Answers

BEST OF FIVE ANSWERS

3.1 B: Vertex deflexed at +1 station

Vertex presentation is a the only presentation in the given choices in which ventouse can be safely applied. Forceps delivery can be performed for after coming head in breech delivery or preterm babies and mento-anterior positions. In infections such as HIV and hepatitis B traumatic delivery should be avoided.

3.2 B: Direct occipito-anterior position

Direct occipito-anterior position is not a prerequisite for instrumental delivery, All the other options in the question should be checked before starting any instrumental delivery. Also the bladder must be emptied.

3.3 B: Addressing psychological and social issues may be important in resolving symptoms

Chronic pelvic pain is so defined if it is > 6 months' duration. Irritable bowel syndrome can be diagnosed based on symptoms. Diagnostic laparoscopy is the second line of investigation after other therapeutic interventions have failed. Combined oral contraceptives and progesterone rather than gonadotrophin releasing hormone should be tried first in endometriosis-associated pain in young women because of better side effect profiles.

Questions on pages 149–158

3.4 C: Ultrasound in the first trimester reduces the induction rates for post-term pregnancy

Induction should be offered after 41 weeks in an uncomplicated pregnancy. A prostaglandin induction increases the risk of scar dehiscence by two to three-fold in a woman with a previous caesarean section and should be monitored with electronic fetal monitoring in all cases. Stretch and sweep is not offered routinely but could be performed prior to formal induction of labour.

3.5 A: Laparoscopic tubal occlusion should only be performed in a hospital with facilities to perform a laparotomy

Sterilisation in not associated with irregular and heavy periods. Diathermy causes more damage to the tubes and is therefore not recommended. Laparoscopic sterilisation is a day case procedure and vasectomy is an easier operation with rates of failure 10 times lower than tubal sterilisation. Therefore it should be routinely offered to couples considering tubal sterilisation.

3.6 E: Heavy painful periods

Fibroids are composed of smooth muscle fibres. Sarcomatous changes are rare and suspected in women with rapidly growing fibroids with symptoms of pain. Pressure symptoms are common with big fibroids. Submucosal fibroids can cause crampy pain and heavy periods. Fibroids are rarely a cause for infertility.

3.7 A: α-Fetoprotein

α-Fetoprotein levels are used for biochemical screening for Down syndrome as part of a maternal serum screening programme. None of the others are used for screening. The triple test screen (second trimester α-fetoprotein, unconjugated oestriol and human chorionic gonadotrophin) has a sensitivity of about 65% with a 5% false positive rate.

3.8 C: Possible need for hysterectomy

Placenta accreta is a possibility in this case. It can cause massive haemorrhage and patient may need a hysterectomy. Other mentioned risks are also there as in any other LSCS.

3.9 C: Active liver disease

Active liver disease is a contraindication for use of progesterone-only pill.

3.10 D: Prescribe oestrogen cream and repeat smear in 2–3 months

This woman has atrophic vaginitis, which can cause problems with smears. Treatment for atrophic vaginitis will improve the cytological picture. However, repeated inadequate smears will need to be investigated in colposcopy clinic.

3.11 A: Cimetidine medication

Cimetidine can be a cause oligozoospermia. Repeat count should be done 3 months after stopping treatment with cimetidine. Hyperthermia, not hypothermia, affects spermatogenesis.

3.12 C: Hospital-based delivery with facilities for electronic fetal monitoring

Routine induction/lower segment caesarean section is not advisable at 37 weeks if there are no complications. Weekly scans and digital cervical examination are not routine practice. Active management of the third stage is practised because of the risk of postpartum haemorrhage.

3.13 D: Pre-eclampsia

Placental insufficiency due to pre-eclampsia is the most likely cause for IUGR. Anaemia can cause asymmetrical IUGR if severe. There is no suggestion of infections in this case (TORCH). Maternal diabetes often leads to macrosomia except in cases of long-standing diabetes with vascular insufficiency.

3.14 B: Urine pregnancy test

Urine pregnancy testing is most important to perform in this case as this student is forgetful. She should be offered other tests if she is at risk for infection (no regular partner, multiple sexual partners etc.). Progesterone alone in form of levonorgestrel is an effective emergency contraception.

3.15 C: Ventricular septal defect

Ventricular septal defect does not remarkably increase the rate of maternal mortality or maternal complications. Maternal mortality is high in Marfan syndrome, obstructive cardiomyopathy, pulmonary hypertension and Eisenmenger syndrome. Mitral and aortic stenoses also have increased risk.

3.16 B: Hypoglycaemia

Hypocalcaemia, not hypercalcaemia, is a complication associated with diabetes. Hypoglycaemia is a known complication in babies of diabetic women. The other problems are not associated with this condition.

3.17 A: Idiopathic

Bladder carcinoma arises from transitional cells, and it is a rare cause for sensory urgency. Urinary tract infection should be initially ruled out in all cases. Idiopathic sensory urgency is more common that that due to bladder stones.

3.18 D: Mirena (levonorgestrel) coil

Progesterone does not help women with fibroids. Mirena, and not the IUCD, will be effective. Iron and folate supplements will help anaemia but not treat the cause.

3.19 C: Vulval carcinoma can occur in about 30% of cases

Involvement of limbs and trunk occurs in approximately 20% of cases. Vulval carcinoma develops in approximately 5% of cases, therefore there is need for follow up.

3.20 D: Egg donation and in vitro fertilisation (IVF)

Premature menopause due to premature ovarian failure occurs in 1–5% of women. It is associated with smoking and women with history in their family. A FSH > 20 suggests no ovarian reserves. She will need egg donation and IVF. She will also be need HRT later to prevent other effects of menopause.

MULTIPLE CHOICE ANSWERS

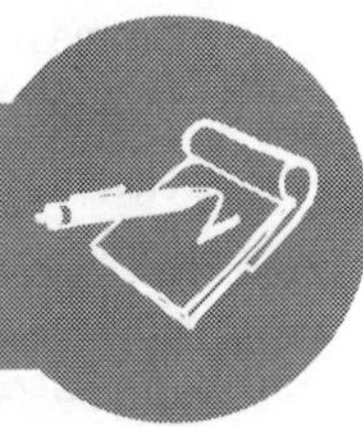

3.21 ACDE

Women who have undergone curative cardiac surgery are at no increased risk, but it is important to get the cardiologist involved in the antenatal care. The remaining conditions are all associated with increased maternal mortality and are grounds for the doctor to consider counselling the woman to avoid pregnancy altogether.

3.22 ACE

Precocious puberty is much more common in girls than in boys and may commence at any age from infancy onwards. Accelerated linear growth is usually its first manifestation. Precocious puberty can be divided into central precocious puberty, ie the hypothalamic pituitary axis is activated, and precocious pseudo-puberty, ie the normal endocrine axis is inactive. True central precocious puberty can be constitutional without any evidence of disorder. This occurs close to the normal time of puberty and is often familial. Idiopathic true precocious puberty is a diagnosis of exclusion and is much more common in girls than in boys. Several neurological disorders can induce early activation of the hypothalamic reproductive axis. Tumours, such as hypothalamic hamartoma and astrocytomas, may also cause this. Previous central nervous insults, such as hydrocephalus, cranial irradiation, infections or skull trauma, may also induce precocious puberty. All cause early release from central inhibition of the endocrine axis and must be considered in the differential diagnosis. Chronic hyperthyroidism is thought to induce central precocious puberty by thyroid stimulating hormone/luteinising hormone overlap. Precocious pseudopuberty is most often caused by oestrogen coming from another source. McCune–Albright syndrome refers to polyostotic fibrous dysplasia characterised by multiple cystic lesions of the skull and long bones, a propensity to fracture, cafe-au-lait skin patches and a predisposition to other endocrine hypersecretion disorders. Some follicular cysts secrete enough oestrogen to induce precocious puberty, but this is not associated with polycystic ovarian syndrome. Granulosa tumours of the ovary may do the same. Some adrenal tumours are also said to feminise rather than virilise, but these are rare. Exogenous estradiol from medications, such as contraceptive pills, or eating meat from oestrogen-treated animals, should not be forgotten as an occasional source of exposure.

3.23 ACD

Congenital varicella zoster is secondary to primary varicella zoster infection, occurring before 20 weeks' gestation. The syndrome includes one or more of the following:

- skin scarring in a dermatomal distribution
- eye defects (microphthalmia, chorioretinitis and cataracts)
- hypoplasia of the limbs
- neurological abnormalities, microcephaly, cortical atrophy, learning disabilities, and dysfunction of bowel and bladder sphincters.

The risk is about 2%, and it does not occur if the primary maternal infection occurs after 20 weeks' gestation.

3.24 BCDE

The definite ways to confirm ovulation are: a pregnancy or picking up the oocyte from the pouch of Douglas. Basal body temperature has a limited role. Other methods of detecting ovarian activity are:

- Changes in cervical mucus with pre-ovulatory cervical mucus clear, acellular and having low viscosity. On the day of ovulation Spinnbarkeit can occur with threads of cervical mucus reaching up to 15–20 cm without breaking.
- Endometrial biopsy demonstrating secretory changes.
- Laparoscopy which can show the corpus luteum.
- Ultrasound scan with sequential ultrasound scanning demonstrating growth of the dominant follicle, rupture and then development of the corpus luteum.
- A rise in the luteinising hormone mid-cycle and a mid-luteal phase progesterone peak are associated with ovulation.

3.25 ACD

Pre-eclampsia is a multisystem disorder having the potential to affect all the systems of the body, including the placenta and the fetus. The prime pathology is an abnormal relationship between the maternal system and the trophoblastic system. Its incidence is greater in diabetic pregnancies, multiple pregnancies and hydatidiform moles. It is interesting that the incidence is lower among women who smoke. It is generally a disease of women in their first pregnancy, but a miscarriage from the same relationship may, in some way, be protective.

3.26 AE

The term 'sex linkage' is virtually synonymous with X linkage; the Y chromosome appears to have few loci apart from those determining the male sex. The only documented Y-linked state is that of the 'hairy pinna'. Congenital ichthyosis is an X-linked disorder associated with a steroid sulphatase deficiency (and hence may be associated with very low oestriol levels in pregnancy). Hurler syndrome is determined by an autosomal recessive gene and achondroplasia by an autosomal dominant gene. Cleft palate, whether or not associated with cleft lip, seems to have a multifactorial inheritance pattern.

3.27 C

Uterine fibroids are benign growths of the myometrium. There are many different forms of treatment and presentation, which usually includes heavy periods and pain, dyspareunia, irregular bleeding and infertility. Medical treatment includes the use of the luteinising hormone-releasing hormone analogue, which reduces the size of the fibroid although it may increase after discontinuation of treatment. Fibroids are dependent on oestrogen and it may be that oestrogen abnormality causes the heavy periods rather than the original theory of increased surface area. Surgical treatment is possible and this may be done with a resectoscope as well as by an open myomectomy. Sarcomatous change is rare. Embolisation of the artery that feeds the fibroid has now been demonstrated to be effective. It does have complications including a risk of hysterectomy. At present it is not suitable for women wanting to maintain their fertility.

3.28 BCDE

Osteoporosis leads to *increased* fragility – read the question! The T score is the bone mineral density in a healthy young adult female population.

3.29 ABCD

Polycystic ovarian syndrome is associated with recurrent spontaneous miscarriage, probably due to the raised basal luteinising hormone. The most common cause of spontaneous abortion is chromosomal abnormalities. These may be recurrent, especially in the older woman and those with a balanced translocation.

3.30 BCDE

The injectable anticoagulant, heparin, is the anticoagulant of choice in pregnancy because it is a large molecule and does not cross the placenta as most oral anticoagulants do. Tetracycline is contraindicated in pregnancy because it crosses the placenta. Adverse effects include deposition in and staining of deciduous teeth and bones, tooth malformation and decrease in linear bone growth. Sulphadimidine rapidly crosses from mother to fetus. If given immediately before delivery there is a theoretical risk of competition between sulphonamides and bilirubin for binding sites on neonatal albumin. Diazepam readily crosses the placenta, which ever route of administration is used, and can cause behavioural problems for many hours after birth if given in late pregnancy or labour. Salicylates cross the placenta and can cause neonatal platelet dysfunction, decreased neonatal factor XII, neonatal haemorrhage and respiratory distress syndrome.

3.31 CE

Cervical eversion is also called cervical ectropion. It is an eversion of the squamocolumnar junction in the lower cervical canal. It gives a florid appearance to the cervix and commonly occurs during adolescence, pregnancy, and while taking the combined oral contraceptive (ie in states of increased oestrogenisation). The term erosion is a misnomer because this does imply an eroded area which would be present in carcinoma. A cervical smear may be indicated before any treatment, but if one is suspicious of cancer of the cervix, a cervical biopsy is the management. Twenty per cent of cervical carcinomas have negative smears and a cervical smear is, therefore, a screening test for premalignant and not malignant disease. Cervical erosions may be asymptomatic, but can cause a variety of symptoms, including chronic vaginal discharge, intermenstrual bleeding and postcoital bleeding. Treatment should only be carried out if the woman is symptomatic.

3.32 ABCE

Neonatal herpes is a severe systemic viral infection with high morbidity. It is most commonly acquired at or near the time of delivery (Royal College of Obstetricians and Gynaecologists Clinical Green Top Guideline). There is no clinical or laboratory evidence of fetal toxicity with aciclovir, and this drug is known to help reduce the duration and severity of symptoms as well as decrease the duration of viral shedding. Caesarean section is recommended for all women presenting with the first episode of genital herpes at the time of delivery.

3.33 DE

The diaphragm is graded in 5 mm sizes and it should be left in position for at least 6 hours after intercourse. In cases of prolapse a good diaphragm fitting is not possible.

3.34 ABCDE

The primary cause of eclampsia is unknown but cerebral vasospasm, ischaemia and oedema are the main effects. Neurological complications include:

- coma
- focal motor deficits
- cortical blindness
- cerebrovascular haemorrhage.

Eclampsia is part of a multisystem disorder and associated complications include:

- HELLP (Haemolysis, elevated liver enzymes and low platelets) – 3%
- Disseminated intravascular coagulation – 3%
- Renal failure – 4%
- Adult respiratory distress syndrome – 3%

3.35 ABE

The risk of the child developing diabetes is thought to be 1–5%. Learning disabilities are uncommon. The blood levels of both calcium and magnesium may fall remarkably during the first 3 days of life if the mother is being treated with insulin; this is thought to be due to delayed development of the baby's parathyroid function.

3.36 ABCDE

Investigation and Management of Endometriosis Guideline 24 (Royal College of Obstetricians and Gynaecologists July, 2000) states that if a woman is not trying to conceive and there is no evidence of a pelvic mass on examination, there may be a role for a therapeutic trial of a combined oral contraceptive (monthly or tricycle) or a progestogen to treat pain symptoms suggestive of endometriosis without performing a diagnostic laparoscopy first. The choice between the combined oral contraceptive, progestogens, danazol and gonadotrophin releasing hormone (GnRH) agonists depends principally on their side-effects profiles because they relieve pain associated with endometriosis equally well. GnRH agonist treatment given for 3 months may be as effective as treatment given for 6 months in relieving endometriosis-associated pain. Using GnRH agonists for greater than 6 months increases the risks of osteoporosis but add-back treatment can be given.

3.37 A

The head may be at the ischial spines when there is a large caput. It is important to perform abdominal palpation at the same time as vaginal examination. A mento-posterior face presentation will not be able to traverse the birth canal because flexion will not occur. Conversely, in a mento-anterior position flexion may result in a subsequent vaginal delivery. The Spalding sign, overlapping of the skull bones due to fetal death in utero, tends to appear by about 3–7 days. Asynclitism is the phenomenon by which the head negotiates the pelvic inlet by a rocking method whereby one parietal bone leads the other. When the head is deflexed, it is not likely to be a vertex, but a malpresentation, eg face or brow.

3.38 ACE

Human chorionic gonadotrophin (hCG) is produced by the placental trophoblast and some other tissues but not by the fetal liver. The level in maternal serum rises rapidly in early pregnancy reaching a peak between 8 and 10 weeks of pregnancy. There is then a rapid reduction to 18 weeks, after which levels remain more or less constant until delivery. hCG almost certainly rescues the corpus luteum from dissolution and promotes placental steroidogenesis. It is also important in the induction of fetal testosterone secretion by Leydig cells in the male fetus. It is suggested that hCG mediates the immunological privilege afforded to the fetus. A variety of gonadal and non-gonadal tumours have been reported to produce hCG, including tumours of the lung, stomach, liver, breast, kidney, pancreas, ovary and testis, carcinoid tumours and lymphomas.

3.39 BCE

Ovulation occurs within 24 hours of the luteinising hormone surge. Oestradiol causes endometrial cell division and this is why it is called proliferation. The proliferative phase can lead to a thickness of the endometrium, up to 6–8 mm in depth. Progesterone causes a withdrawal bleed on an oestrogen-primed endometrium. It is, therefore, not the cessation of oestrogen production, but cessation of progesterone production. Trophoblastic human chorionic gonadotrophin maintains the life of the corpus luteum which otherwise has a limited lifespan of 12–16 days, thus preventing the withdrawal bleed.

3.40 None correct

The incidence of endometrial carcinoma in women aged between 30 and 34 is 0.66 per 100 000 women. Endometrial carcinoma is associated with unopposed oestrogens. The incidence is in the order of 6% after 5 years' use of unopposed oestrogens, rising to 22% after 10 years. As it is usually detected early, with postmenopausal bleeding or irregular bleeding, the prognosis is good and the treatment is generally surgery followed by radiotherapy in some cases. Endometrial carcinoma is not usually diagnosed by ultrasound scanning; a thick endometrium in a woman who is postmenopausal is suggestive of it, but not diagnostic.

3.41 ABCD

	Apgar scores		
	0	1	2
Heart rate	Absent	< 100 bpm	> 100 bpm
Respiratory effort	Absent	Weak, irregular	Strong cry
Muscle tone	Limp	Some limb flexion	Active motion
Reflex irritability response on suctioning the pharynx	No	Grimace	Cough or cry
Colour	Pale/overall cyanosis	Peripherally blue, centrally pink	Pink all over

3.42 D

The incidence of ectopic pregnancy is increased to about 3% in conceptions following in vitro fertilisation or gamete intrafallopian transfer. Suspicion should be raised in any woman who misses a period and easy access to β-human chorionic gonadotrophin pregnancy testing units is essential. The different forms of surgical treatment available are laparoscopic removal and salpingostomy, but salpingectomy may be done. Medical treatment has been, and still is, under investigation, including injection of methotrexate into the sac.

3.43 CDE

Open neural tissue in the fetus will result in the passage of fetal proteins into the maternal circulation. Spina bifida occulta is a closed lesion, so this will not cause a rise in the α-fetoprotein level. Down syndrome may be associated with low serum levels of α-fetoprotein. Threatened abortion may result in fetal–maternal transfusion, hence the presence of fetal blood will raise maternal serum α-fetoprotein. Multiple pregnancy will cause a rise in α-fetoprotein – the exact mechanism of this is unknown, but it presumably reflects the increased amount of fetal tissue.

3.44 CDE

Bacterial vaginosis is the most common infective cause of vaginitis, being twice as common as *Candida* infection. It is a microbial disease due to decrease in the *Lactobacillus* species and an increase in anaerobic bacteria. The incidence is high in lesbians. For diagnosis three of the following four features should be present:

- Clue cells
- Homogeneous discharge adherent to vagina walls
- pH in vagina greater than 4.5
- Fishy smell, especially if potassium hydroxide added.

It is asymptomatic in 50% of cases. Symptoms include excessive white-grey discharge and a noticeable odour following sexual intercourse.

3.45 ABDE

The typical female pelvis in Caucasian women has a brim which is slightly wider in its transverse than its anteroposterior diameter (gynaecoid), the true obstetric conjugate being 11–12 cm and the transverse 13 cm. The cavity has the contours of a curved cylinder rather than a funnel, the side walls being approximately parallel. The greater sciatic notch is usually greater than 90° and the subpubic angle should also approximate to a right angle.

3.46 ABC

Fetal lung alveoli are lined by a group of phospholipids known collectively as surfactant, which prevent collapse of the alveoli during respiration by reducing surface tension. The predominant phospholipid is phosphatidyl choline (lecithin) and a surge in its production occurs at around 35 weeks' gestation in normal pregnancy, promoted by glucocorticoids. Fetal lung maturity seems to be accelerated in some cases of pre-eclampsia, learning disabilities and premature rupture of the membranes and is delayed in diabetes mellitus. α-Fetoprotein is of no relevance to pulmonary maturity.

3.47 BCE

Cystadenoma, granulosa cell tumour and teratoma may all occur in the ovary, being derived from neoplastic growth in epithelial, sex cord and germ cell structures, respectively. Nephroblastoma and neuroblastoma are developmental tumours of kidney and nerve tissue, respectively, occurring almost exclusively in early childhood and generally showing a sarcomatous appearance.

3.48 E

Amniocentesis, if performed under ultrasound guidance, is associated with a pregnancy loss of about 1:200. It does not seem that the position of the placenta increases the risk of placental wastage. Amniocentesis is useful to diagnose genetic disease and it is the ultrasound scan that is the diagnostic for open neural tube defects. It is interesting that 2% of amniotic fluid samples fail to culture and these have a higher association with a congenital abnormality.

3.49 AC

Chlamydia, although it has an intracellular existence, differs from a virus by its large size, complex cellular envelope and possession of both RNA and DNA. The treatment of choice is tetracycline, such as doxycycline, but if the woman is pregnant then erythromycin should be used. The common heat-stable antigen may be used as an enzyme-linked method of detection. *Chlamydia* may also be detected by direct staining smears. Fitz–Hugh–Curtis syndrome is a syndrome of fibrinous perihepatitis associated with pelvic peritonitis. The woman may present with upper abdominal pain and tubal damage can occur. Therefore, infertility is a long-term sequela.

3.50 ABE

PPH is a potentially life-threatening complication of both vaginal and caesarean deliveries. PPH is defined as blood loss greater than 500 ml during delivery. PPH can be divided into:

- Primary PPH that occurs within 24 hours after delivery.
- Secondary PPH that occurs 24 hours to 6 weeks after delivery.

The exact incidence of PPH is difficult to determine. PPH occurs in 2–8% of deliveries. Secondary PPH occurs in approximately 1% of all deliveries. The most frequent cause of PPH is uterine atony (90%). Other causes are: lacerations of the cervix and/or vagina, retained placenta, disorders of coagulation and thrombocytopenia, uterine inversion and rupture uterus. Risk factors include: prolonged labour, pre-eclampsia, previous PPH, multiple gestation, coagulation abnormalities, forceps or ventouse delivery, multiparity (20-fold increase in risk) and polyhydramnios.

3.51 ACDE

Nausea and vomiting are the most frequent and perhaps the most troublesome symptoms of early pregnancy. The exact aetiology is unknown and the condition is usually self-limiting. Antihistamines are better than a placebo and are generally considered to be safe during pregnancy. Sometimes antihistamines can cause troublesome side-effects, including drowsiness and blurring of vision. It is important to remember that epigastric pain and late onset of nausea and vomiting may be a presenting feature of pre-eclampsia, specifically HELLP syndrome. Increased trophoblastic tissue with a hydatidiform mole may give exaggerated signs of pregnancy; this may be not only excessive nausea and vomiting but also early pre-eclampsia. It is important to do an ultrasound scan as part of the management of a woman with nausea and vomiting.

3.52 ABCDE

Chromosome abnormalities, particularly of the X chromosome, can occur. X-chromosome mosaicisms are the most common abnormality. In Turner syndrome (45XO) accelerated follicular loss causes ovarian failure. Familial premature ovarian failure has been associated with fragile X permutations. Women with Down syndrome also have premature menopause. Autoimmune diseases including hypothyroidism, Addison's disease and diabetes may be associated with premature ovarian failure. The metabolic disease galactosaemia is associated with premature ovarian failure. Hysterectomy with conservation of the ovaries can induce ovarian failure. In these women it is advisable to perform annual follicle-stimulating hormone measurements, especially in those who have had a hysterectomy before the age of 40. Infection, including mumps and tuberculosis, may be associated with premature ovarian failure.

3.53 BDE

Basal body temperature measurement is a poor method for ovulation detection and has a limited role (if any) in the investigation of an infertile woman. Basal body temperature often drops transiently by 0.1–0.2 °C around the time of ovulation followed by a sustained rise of 0.5–1.0 °C which is maintained throughout the luteal phase. The plasma luteinising hormone surges to a peak around 12 hours before ovulation and falls progressively during the luteal phase. Plasma progesterone secretion by the corpus luteum increases to a peak around 7–8 days after ovulation and, as a result, the endometrium undergoes a secretory change and cervical mucus becomes more scanty, viscid and cellular.

3.54 ACD

A woman with antepartum haemorrhage requires hospital assessment and vaginal examination should not be performed until the placental site is known. In placental abruption, vaginal blood loss is not an accurate indication of severity.

3.55 E

When counselling a patient for sterilisation the acronym FILMVE should be used to ascertained the following:

- F – The woman knows the failure rate is about 1:500
- I – The woman has been fully informed that it is irreversible. If she thinks it is reversible then it is contraindicated
- L – The woman is aware that it is done by the laparoscopic method, although it may be necessary to do a mini-laparotomy if the tubes are not visible
- M – The woman knows that the menses should not be affected; however, if she has been on the pill before being sterilised then coming off the pill may be associated with heavy periods which is endogenous rather than exogenous in relation.
- V – Her partner has thought about vasectomy.
- E – Ectopic pregnancy is a risk when sterilisation failure occurs.

3.56 AD

With increasing maternal age there is an increase in chromosomal abnormalities associated with the increasing age of the oocytes. There is also an increase in the background luteinising hormone. Both of the above may predispose to an increase in miscarriage.

3.57 BCD

Genital herpes is usually caused by herpes virus hominis type II, whereas ordinary lip herpes is caused by herpes virus hominis type I. Penicillin and other treponemicidal drugs should *not* be given as they may confuse the diagnosis of coincidental syphilis.

3.58 ADE

Female sterilisation is the most commonly used method of contraception in the age group of 40–49 years. Vasectomy is more popular in younger couples. Healthy, normal body mass index, non-smoking women with no cardiovascular risk factors may continue to use the low-dose combined oral contraceptive until the age of 50 years. Women who smoke are best advised to stop at the age of 35 years. The progestogen-only pill is an excellent form of contraception for the older woman as it has few contraindications, and is highly effective in this group if taken in the correct way. Poor cycle control is a major disadvantage. Emergency contraception can be used in this group. The only contraindication is migraine at presentation in a woman with a history of migraine with aura. The progestogen-only method has been shown to cause less nausea and vomiting than the combined method and to have improved efficacy.

3.59 AB

Definitions like these can be difficult as books give subtly different answers. Primary amenorrhoea is defined as no menstruation by 14 years of age with growth failure or absence of secondary sexual characteristics, ie breast development and pubic hair growth; or no menstruation by 16 years of age when growth and sexual development are normal. Secondary amenorrhoea is defined as the absence of menses for 6 months in a previously menstruating woman. The climacteric is the time when a woman changes from being able to reproduce to being unable to reproduce and puberty is the opposite, ie the time when a woman becomes able to sexually reproduce. The last menstrual period is the menopause and the first menstrual period is the menarche. Dysmenorrhoea can be primary or secondary. Primary dysmenorrhoea is defined as pain which begins on the first day of menstruation but reduces as menstruation proceeds. It usually occurs in the younger woman and is associated with ovulation. Secondary dysmenorrhoea is pain beginning 1–5 days before the onset of menstruation which is relieved by menstruation. It is usually associated with pathology in the older woman. Such pathology includes endometriosis, fibroids and pelvic inflammatory disease. It may also be associated with the intrauterine contraceptive device.

3.60 BC

Thrombosis and thromboembolism remain the **main direct cause** of maternal death. Although they account for 25-30% of all direct maternal deaths, the rate has fallen since the last Report.

Hypertensive disease of pregnancy is the 3rd leading cause of direct deaths (haemorrhage is 2nd)

Deaths in early pregnancy include several causes. The largest number is due to ectopic pregnancy.

The Confidential Enquiries into Maternal Deaths in the United Kingdom (2000-2002), Executive Summary and Key Recommendations, CEMACH website; http://www.cemach.org.uk

EXTENDED MATCHING QUESTIONS ANSWERS

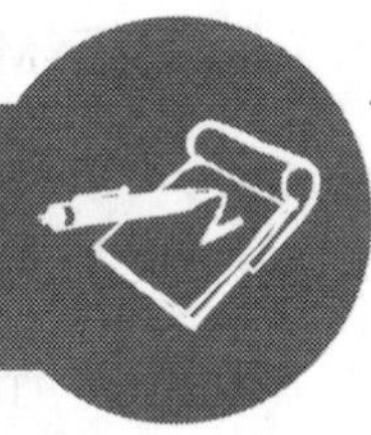

20 Questions: Time allowed 30 minutes. Please give the single most appropriate answer from the list of alternatives.

THEME: GENETICS

3.61 D 1 in 4 chance. If there is an affected child the parents are both carriers of the cystic fibrosis gene. The inheritance is autosomal recessive therefore offspring will be: 1 in 4 will have cystic fibrosis, 2 in 4 unaffected carriers and 1 in 4 unaffected and not a carrier.

3.62 B 1 in 2 males will be affected (X-linked recessive inheritance).

3.63 F No pattern of inheritance. Affected male to son transmission does not occur in a disease with X-linked recessive inheritance.

THEME: PRENATAL DIAGNOSIS

3.64 F 60–70%

3.65 G > 90%

3.66 E 30–40%

Questions on pages 175–184

THEME: MISCARRIAGE

3.67 D Missed miscarriage (blighted ovum). A gestational sac of > 20 mm with no fetal pole is diagnostic.

3.68 F Threatened miscarriage.

3.69 B Incomplete miscarriage.

THEME: CONTRACEPTION

3.70 E Levonelle and condoms. Levonelle is 90% effective as an emergency contraception if taken within 24 hours of unprotected intercourse. Offer screening for sexually transmitted infections, do a pregnancy test and provide condoms.

3.71 C Implanon. This does not need to be remembered every day and stays for 3 years. Also it can be inserted under anaesthesia if the patient is going for a surgical termination of pregnancy.

3.72 G Mirena coil. This coil is as effective as female sterilisation and stays for 5 years.

THEME: GYNAECOLOGICAL CANCER

3.73 F Tamoxifen. Unopposed oestrogen action on the endometrium is associated with an increased risk of endometrial cancer.

3.74 C Human papilloma virus especially subtypes 16, 18 are oncogenic and cause high-grade cervical intraepithelial neoplasia lesions and cancer of the cervix.

3.75 A BRCA1 and BRCA2 gene mutations are linked with cancer of the breast and ovary.

THEME: ABDOMINAL PAIN IN PREGNANCY

3.76 E Placental abruption. The positive Kleihauer test indicates that there has been a placental problem leading to loss of fetal blood into the maternal circulation. Vaginal bleeding does not occur in a concealed abruption.

3.77 B Appendicitis can be difficult to diagnose in later pregnancy. The pain from a torsion of an ovarian cyst is typically intermittent and that of appendicitis is constant. Ultrasound or clinical identification of a mass confirms presence of an ovarian mass.

3.78 G Round ligament tendinitis can be subtle. Palpation of the tender round ligaments is helpful.

THEME: PRETERM RUPTURE OF MEMBRANES

3.79 G Erythromycin orally. The pregnancy will be treated conservatively and oral erythromycin prescribed.

3.80 E Conservative management with no medication. If labour progresses there will be no suppression due to the possibility of intrauterine infection. If labour does not progress there is no indication to augment if the fetus is well.

3.81 G Erythromycin orally. The footling breech presentation will dictate the mode of delivery (ie caesarean section) when delivery occurs but conservative management will be undertaken in the first instance.

THEME: ANAESTHESIA IN OBSTETRICS

3.82 E Pethidine (intramuscular). Epidural and spinal analgesia are contraindicated with placental abruption as there is a risk of coagulopathy. The other forms of pain relief are probably not sufficient for active labour.

3.83 A Epidural anaesthesia. Opiates should be avoided in this case but good analgesia is essential. Regional techniques are indicated and an epidural preferred to a spinal because of the duration of effect and the ability to repeat the block via an epidural catheter.

3.84 F Spinal anaesthesia is preferred over a general or epidural. Spinal anaesthesia provides a more predictable effect than an epidural and is safer for the mother than a general anaesthetic.

THEME: GENERAL GYNAECOLOGY

3.85 B This is a classic presentation of endometriosis.

3.86 A Chronic pelvic inflammatory disease – this is suggested by a vaginal discharge associated with chronic pelvic pain and subfertility from tubal damage.

3.87 D Pelvic adhesions. This is suggested by the history of multiple abdominal surgery and chronic pelvic pain.

THEME: GENERAL GYNAECOLOGY

3.88 F Turner syndrome – a webbed neck in association with primary amenorrhoea is characteristic.

3.89 B Meigs syndrome – The triad is characteristic.

3.90 D Polycystic ovary syndrome is associated with oligomenorrhoea and infertility.

Practice Paper 4
Questions

BEST OF FIVE QUESTIONS

PAPER 4 BOFS

20 Questions: Time allowed 30 minutes. Please give the single most appropriate answer from the list of alternatives.

4.1 A woman has a history of three miscarriages between 12 and 20 weeks. Which one of the following is the most likely cause for her poor obstetric history.

- A Müllerian duct anomaly
- B *Toxoplasma gondii* infection
- C Malaria
- D Hepatitis B
- E Asthma

4.2 For which one of the following clinical situations is colposcopy not the best next line of investigation?

- A More than one consecutive smear result showing cervical intraepithelial neoplasia (CIN) 1
- B CIN II smear result
- C CIN III smear result
- D Cervical growth
- E Two or more borderline smears

Answers on pages 255–258

4.3 A 30-year-old pregnant woman with a previous stillbirth is diagnosed as having antiphospholipid antibody syndrome. You are counselling her about the risk associated with the disease. Which one of the following is a problem that probably occurs with the same frequency as in the general population?

- A Recurrent miscarriage
- B Placental abruption
- C Intrauterine growth restriction (IUGR)
- D Increased risk of congenital malformation
- E Venous thrombosis

4.4 Which one of the following is the most appropriate feature of an imperforate hymen?

- A It is usually identified at birth
- B It may lead in haematosalpinx and infertility
- C It is frequently associated with renal anomalies
- D Is found in association with a bicornuate uterus
- E It requires McIndoe reconstructive surgery

4.5 A G5 P4 has just delivered her placenta. She bleeds approximately 1 litre due to atonic uterus. You have given her oxytocics and started fluids. A midwife is massaging her uterus which keeps relaxing. Which one of the following options is the most appropriate next step in her management?

- A Check placenta and membranes for completeness.
- B Hysterectomy
- C Internal iliac artery ligation
- D Blood transfusion
- E Pack uterus with gauze

4.6 An overweight woman with irregular periods presents with hirsutism. Which one of the following is the most likely cause for her hirsutism?

- A Thyroid disease
- B Acromegaly
- C Bulimia
- D Cushing syndrome
- E Polycystic ovarian disease

4.7 A woman who delivered 4 days ago is complaining of poor lactation. Which one of the following medications is best avoided for her as she is keen to breast feed?

- A Cimetidine
- B Opiates
- C Prochlorperazine
- D Metaclopromide
- E Cabergoline

4.8 A woman is requesting epidural anaesthesia in the first stage of labour. Which one of the following situations is an indication for epidural anaesthesia?

- A Severe aortic stenosis
- B Intravenous opiate misuse
- C Coagulopathy
- D Severe thrombocytopenia
- E Localised or systemic sepsis

4.9 A primigravida who is non-immune to rubella comes in contact with it in the first trimester of her pregnancy. Which one of the following is not likely to be a feature of congenital rubella infection in the baby?

A Hydrocephalus

B Thrombocytopenia

C Deafness

D Patent ductus arteriosus

E Cataract

4.10 A pregnant woman who had an antenatal ultrasound suggestive of a diaphragmatic hernia has just delivered. Which one of the following represents the best possible management option for the neonate?

A Give the baby to the mother

B Artificial ventilation with Ambu bag

C Intranasal catheter and ventilation

D IV cannulation + nasogastric tube

E Early intubation + nasogastric tube

4.11 You are asked to review a cardiotocograph for a primigravida at 35 weeks of pregnancy. She ruptured her membranes 24 hours ago. The baseline is around 105 with normal variability. Which one of the following is a likely cause?

- A Extreme prematurity
- B Maternal dehydration
- C Maternal hyperthermia
- D Maternal hyperthyroidism on treatment
- E Chorioamnionitis

4.12 A diabetic woman with body mass index of 40 kg/m^2 has been prepared for forceps delivery following a prolonged second stage of labour. You should be ready to deal with which one of the most likely complications in this case?

- A Scalp injury to baby
- B Uterine rupture
- C Shoulder dystocia
- D APH (Acute partum haemorrhage)
- E Retained placenta

4.13 With regard to external cephalic version (ECV) for breech presentation, which one of the following statements is the best description of an aspect of ECV?

- A Use of tocolysis reduces complications
- B Should be performed at 33 weeks
- C Should be performed in theatre
- D If performed at term may reduce the incidence of operative delivery
- E Fetal death is a common complication

4.14 A woman has gestational diabetes and needed insulin for control of her blood sugar. Which one of the following is the most appropriate management plan for her after delivery?

- A To continue half dose of insulin after delivery
- B Oral hypoglycaemic medications
- C Continue same dose of insulin
- D Stop insulin, glucose tolerance test 6 weeks later
- E Reassure and discharge

4.15 A 30-year-old woman has a body mass index of 45 kg/m^2 and complains of oligomenorrhoea. You are motivating her to lose weight. Weight loss is unlikely to help her in reducing her chances of developing which one of the following problems?

A Endometrial carcinoma

B Infertility

C Breast cancer

D Menopausal symptoms

E Urinary dysfunction

4.16 A 15-year-old girl has recently immigrated from Africa. She has a body mass index of 16 kg/m^2. Breast development is stage 2 Tanner and she has primary amenorrhoea. What is the most likely cause for her late menarche?

A McCune–Albright syndrome

B Ovarian tumour

C Brain trauma

D Undernutrition

E Cerebral tumours

4.17 A 50-year-old menopausal woman suffers from hot flushes and sweating. Which one of the following is the best possible treatment option for her?

A Oestrogen patches

B Tibolone

C Oestrogen orally

D Oestrogen + progesterone

E Raloxifene

4.18 A 50-year-old women presents with bone pains, and bone densitometry suggests osteoporosis. Which one of the following conditions is most unlikely to contribute to bone loss?

A Diabetes mellitus

B Anticonvulsant therapy

C Gastrectomy

D Hypoparathyroidism

E Chronic neurological disease

4.19 A primipara smokes 20 cigarettes a day. She conceives after in vitro fertilisation with a twin gestation. She is anxious as her mother died of eclampsia. Which one of the following factors is unlikely to increase her risk of pre-eclampsia?

A Primiparity

B Obesity

C Smoking

D Twin gestation

E Positive family history

4.20 An 8-week pregnant primipara is admitted with epigastric pain, vomiting and weight loss of 3 kg over 2 weeks. Which one of the following conditions is most likely to be responsible for her problems?

A Diabetic ketoacidosis

B Pancreatitis

C Drug-induced vomiting

D Thyrotoxicosis

E Hyperemesis gravidarum

MULTIPLE CHOICE QUESTIONS

40 Questions: Time allowed 1½ hours. Indicate your answers clearly by putting a tick against the correct or true options and a cross against the incorrect or false options. (The section on answers in this book lists the correct (true) options.)

4.21 The following statements about starting combined oral contraceptives (COC) is/are true:

- A Starting on day 1 of menstruation extra precautions are required for 7 days
- B If post partum and not lactating COC can be started on day 21
- C During lactation the COC can be started after 49 days
- D After an induced early abortion or miscarriage a COC can be started the next day
- E The COC can be started after a progestogen-only pill on the first day of a period and no extra precautions are required

4.22 Recognised causes of jaundice in the newborn include:

- A A cephalohaematoma following a ventouse delivery
- B Physiological causes that occur around day 7
- C Infection
- D Rhesus incompatibility
- E Hypothyroidism with jaundice occurring in the first 2 days

Answers on pages 259–271

4.23 In breech presentation:

- A The perinatal morbidity is greater in the extended than in the flexed type
- B Meconium is a reliable indicator of fetal distress
- C Variable decelerations of fetal heart rate is a likely finding during intrapartum monitoring
- D Breech extraction is the method of choice for a safe vaginal delivery
- E Obstetric forceps are not necessary in multiparous women

4.24 Which of the drug–side-effect combinations listed below are correct?

- A Oestrogens – weight gain
- B Aciclovir – rise in bilirubin and liver enzymes
- C Fluconazole – nausea and abdominal discomfort
- D Bromocriptine – hypertension
- E Danazol – dry skin

4.25 Risk factors for pre-eclampsia include:

- A Obesity
- B Previous severe pre-eclampsia
- C Underweight and short stature
- D Age between 25 and 35 years
- E Chronic renal disease

4.26 The following statements about hydatidiform mole is/are correct:

A There is a decreased incidence with increasing age

B It may present with pre-eclampsia

C It gives a typical ultrasound appearance

D It is monitored after evacuation by urinary oestriol levels

E It is treated by methotrexate

4.27 With regard to ovarian cancer:

A Most women with early-stage cancer of the ovary do not have any symptoms

B Ovarian cancer may present as postmenopausal bleeding

C The incidence increases with age to peak in the 40–50-year age group

D Normal CA125 levels exclude ovarian cancer

E CA125 may increase in pelvic inflammatory disease

4.28 With regard to *Why Mothers Die?* in comparison with the 1997–1999 report, the overall findings in the 2000–2002 report showed:

A More deaths due to indirect causes than direct causes in 2000–2002

B Mortality rate for eclampsia/pre-eclampsia was markedly lower during 2000–2002 than in 1997–1999

C Maternal mortality rates were higher in socially disadvantaged, late bookers, substance misusers and women suffering domestic violence

D Mortality rates due to haemorrhage doubled since 1997–1999

E Most common cause of indirect death remains thromboembolism

4.29 If a pregnant woman comes into contact with rubella:

A The majority of women will have an abnormal fetus

B A blood test taken immediately showing IgG antibodies means the fetus will not be affected

C The baby may have high-tone deafness

D Gammaglobulin should be given as soon as possible

E The highest risk of fetal damage is at 4 weeks' gestation

4.30 Predisposing factors for uterovaginal prolapse include:

- A High parity
- B The menopause
- C Ascites
- D Previous treatment with large loop excision of transformation zone (LLETZ)
- E Chronic cough

4.31 With regard to gynaecological malignancies:

- A Endometrial carcinoma spreads to lymphatics less readily than cervical carcinoma
- B Radiotherapy is the treatment of choice for a malignant pyometra
- C In a Wertheim hysterectomy the lower third of the vagina is excised
- D The ovaries may be conserved in the surgical treatment of carcinoma of the corpus uteri
- E Renal failure is a common cause of death in cervical carcinoma

4.32 The following statements about infection in pregnancy is/are true:

- A Rubella is an RNA virus
- B Toxoplasmosis can be treated by spiramycin
- C Congenital varicella syndrome occurs in about 1:1000 deliveries
- D Listeriosis is associated with spontaneous miscarriage
- E Listeriosis can be treated by ampicillin

4.33 Dilatation and curettage (D&C):

- A Was performed at a rate of 71.1/1000 women in 1989–1990
- B Is being replaced by outpatient procedures
- C Samples all the endometrium
- D Has a 5% false-negative rate
- E Is associated with uterine perforation

4.34 Treatment of acute vulvovaginal candidiasis includes:

- A Topical clotrimazole 1%
- B Topical econazole 1%
- C Topical miconazole 2%
- D Oral fluconazole 150 mg stat
- E Itraconazole 200 mg two times for 1 day

4.35 Constipation during pregnancy:

- A Can be treated with magnesium salts during pregnancy
- B Can be treated with dioctyl sodium sulphosuccinate during pregnancy
- C Can be prevented by increasing the amount of fibre in the diet
- D Is associated with a decrease in gut motility
- E Is particularly bad in the first trimester of pregnancy

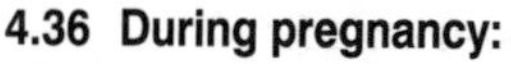

4.36 During pregnancy:

- A Glycosuria is an effective test of carbohydrate intolerance
- B Fasting plasma glucose concentration is decreased
- C Fasting plasma insulin concentration is decreased
- D The oral glucose tolerance test alters with advancing gestation
- E 2 hours after an oral glucose load, plasma insulin concentration should have returned to fasting levels

4.37 An 18-year-old woman complains of never having had a period. She has normal breast development and is 157 cm in height. Secondary sexual development commenced 3 years previously. Chromosomal analysis is normal and blood tests indicate serum luteinising hormone level of 10.6 IU/l, and serum follicle-stimulating hormone level of 4.6 IU/l. Possible explanations include:

- A Androgen insensitivity syndrome
- B Polycystic ovarian disease
- C Constitutional delayed puberty
- D Primary ovarian failure
- E Imperforate hymen

4.38 Common causes of meningitis in the newborn include:

- A *Neisseria meningitidis*
- B *Haemophilus influenzae*
- C *Escherichia coli*
- D Group B streptococci
- E Pneumococci

4.39 Key findings of the 2000–2002 Confidential Enquiries into Maternal And Child Health (CEMACH) report include:

- A Overall maternal mortality rate for UK in 2000–2002 was 13/10 000
- B There was an increase in deaths due to haemorrhage
- C There was a decrease in deaths due to anaesthesia
- D Women living in deprived areas have 45% higher death rates
- E 35% of all women who died were obese

4.40 Advantages of copper-containing intrauterine contraceptive devices include:

- A They are effective
- B They are reversible
- C They are cheap
- D They reduce menstrual blood loss
- E There are no known unwanted systemic effects

4.41 Principles of antenatal care include:

- A Dietary advice should focus on a well-balanced and varied diet, such as raw meat and soft cheeses
- B Vigorous exercise should be limited to an hour daily
- C Pelvic floor exercises should be included in all antenatal exercise programmes
- D A minimum of four antenatal visits is recommended for a woman with a normal pregnancy
- E Early antenatal care is important in the prevention and treatment of anaemia

4.42 Pruritus vulvae:

- A Is the same as vulvodynia
- B Can be caused by lichen sclerosus
- C Is experienced by 1% of women worldwide
- D Is contributed to by glycosuria and diabetes
- E Occurs as a result of purulent and mucopurulent vaginal discharge in 20% of cases

4.43 Vulvodynia:

- A Is known as vulvar vestibulitis syndrome
- B Is defined as acute vulval pain
- C Often occurs in a vagina that shows no abnormalities
- D Occurs only on provocation, such as with attempted vaginal penetration for sexual intercourse
- E Has a prevalence as high as 15%

4.44 With regard to induction of labour:

- A It can be conducted on an antenatal ward
- B Cardiotocogram should be performed prior to induction of labour
- C Prolonged use of maternal facial oxygen treatment should be used whenever needed
- D Continuous cardiotocography should not be used with induction of labour with oxytocin
- E Women with uncomplicated pregnancies should be offered induction of labour prior to 41 weeks

4.45 With regard to a singleton pregnancy:

- A Softening of the lower third of the vagina, the Hegar sign, occurs around 6 weeks
- B Physical signs during the first trimester are reliable predictors of pregnancy
- C Average duration of pregnancy is 266 days from the date of ovulation
- D The uterus begins to enlarge 8 weeks after implantation
- E Half of pregnant women will experience nausea and vomiting in the first trimester

4.46 With regard to fertilisation and implantation:

A Fertilisation occurs 6 hours after ovulation

B Implantation usually occurs within about 48 hours of ovulation

C Fertilisation usually occurs in the ampulla

D The most common site of abnormal implantation is in the uterine tube

E Spermatogenesis occurs in the seminiferous tubules of testes and begins at the time of birth

4.47 With regard to β-human chorionic gonadotrophin (β-hCG):

A Trophoblastic cells produce hCG

B hCG levels double every 1.3–2 days

C Modern urine pregnancy tests can detect hCG concentrations as low as 0.5 mIU/ml

D Urine pregnancy tests can be positive 3 days after implantation

E Radioimmunoassay techniques for measuring serum β-hCG can detect levels as low as 2 mIU/ml

4.48 Risk factors for ectopic pregnancy include:

A Previous history of pelvic inflammatory disease

B Previous tubal surgery

C Previous ectopic pregnancy

D Intrauterine contraceptive device (coil) in situ

E In vitro fertilisation (IVF) or assisted fertilisation

4.49 Serum human chorionic gonadotrophin (hCG):

- A Can be positive within 7–10 days of conception
- B Doubles approximately every 48 hours in 85% of normal intrauterine pregnancies of 4–6 weeks
- C Rises < 66% in 48 hours in more than 80% of ectopic pregnancies
- D At levels of 500 IU/l should normally indicate a visible intrauterine sac
- E May also be increased with certain types of ovarian tumours and testicular tumours

4.50 Risk factors for cord prolapse include:

- A Multiple pregnancy
- B Breech presentation
- C Transverse and oblique lie
- D Polyhydramnios
- E Preterm labour

4.51 With regard to cervical cancer screening in UK:

- A It is started at 20 years of age in sexually active women
- B It is recommended every 3 years
- C It is recommended every 5 years after 50 years of age until 65 years
- D A patient with moderate dyskaryosis need referral for colposcopy
- E An Ayres spatula should be used

4.52 With regard to amenorrhoea the following statements is/are true:

A Primary amenorrhoea is defined as absence of menstruation by 14 years of age in the presence of development of secondary sexual characteristics

B Women who undergo premature ovarian failure (secondary amenorrhoea) before 40 years should all have chromosomal analysis

C Testicular feminisation patients should be treated with anti-androgens

D Laparoscopic biopsy of the ovary should be performed to reach a diagnosis of premature ovarian failure

E If a patient bleeds on progesterone challenge a diagnosis of anovulation should be considered

4.53 Which of the statements given below about infertility is/are true?

A Infertility affects about 10% of couples

B 35% of cases are due to male factors while 65% are due to female factors

C Polycystic ovarian syndrome (PCOS) is the commonest cause of female infertility

D 10% of unexplained infertility patients will achieve pregnancy in 3 years of conservative treatment

E Routine hysteroscopy should be done in infertile women to rule out uterine causes of infertility

4.54 Risk factors for placental abruption include:

A Previous abruption

B Rapid uterine decompression

C Increasing maternal age

D Previous uterine surgery

E Chronic chorioamnionitis

4.55 Maternal risks associated with repeat elective caesarean section include:

A Increased risk of uterine rupture

B Increased risk of placenta praevia and accreta in subsequent pregnancy

C Increased risk of perineal trauma

D Increased hospital stay

E Slight increase in subfertility

4.56 The following parameters are used for Apgar score:

A Blood pressure

B Heart rate

C Breathing

D Reflex response

E Passage of meconium

4.57 The following cannot cause postpartum cardiovascular collapse:

A Uterine inversion

B Amniotic fluid embolism

C Cardiac arrhythmia

D Hypothyroidism

E Pulmonary embolism

4.58 The following are risk factors for uterovaginal prolapse:

A Menopause

B Smoking

C Constipation

D African-Caribbean origin

E Childbirth

4.59 Factors related to dyspareunia are:

A Arousal problems

B Essential vulvodynia

C Episiotomy

D Intrauterine contraceptive device (IUCD)

E Subtotal hysterectomy

4.60 Which of the statements regarding vulvovaginal candidiasis is/are true?

A Treatment is not warranted in asymptomatic cases

B Topical and oral treatment are equally effective

C Oral treatment with imidazoles should be avoided in pregnancy

D Partner treatment is effective for recurrent infection

E It is recurrent in 5% cases

EXTENDED MATCHING QUESTIONS

30 Questions: Time allowed 1 hour.

THEME: MATERNAL MORTALITY

A Amniotic fluid embolism
B Anaesthetic related
C Cancer
D Cardiac disease
E Ectopic pregnancy
F Haemorrhage
G Pre-eclampsia/eclampsia
H Psychiatric causes
I Thromboembolism

Instructions: With regard to the report into the confidential enquiries into maternal deaths in the United Kingdom 2000–2002, from the list above choose the most appropriate answer to the following questions about maternal deaths. Each option can be used once, more than once or not at all.

4.61 What was the most common cause of direct deaths?

4.62 What was the most common cause of indirect deaths?

4.63 If maternal deaths up to 1 year after delivery are included what is the leading cause?

Answers on pages 273–276

THEME: VAGINAL BIRTH AFTER CAESAREAN SECTION

A Augmentation of labour with an oxytocin infusion
B Elective repeat caesarean section
C Induction of labour with prostaglandin
D Previous classic caesarean section
E Previous vaginal delivery
F Twin pregnancy in current pregnancy
G Two previous lower segment caesarean sections

Instructions: From the list above choose the best association that applies to a woman requesting a trial of vaginal delivery after a caesarean section. Each option can be used once, more than once or not at all.

4.64 The condition representing a contraindication to vaginal delivery after a previous caesarean section.

4.65 The condition representing the lowest risk for uterine rupture.

4.66 The condition representing the most favourable condition for a successful vaginal delivery.

THEME: POSTNATAL PROBLEMS

A Chest infection
B Deep venous thrombosis
C Endometritis
D Mastitis
E Pelvic haematoma
F Septic pelvic thrombophlebitis
G Urinary tract infection
H Wound infection

Instructions: From the list above choose the most likely diagnosis for each clinical scenario given below. Each option can be used once, more than once or not at all.

4.67 A woman on day 3 post caesarean section, feeling unwell with a pyrexia, rigors and normal lochia.

4.68 A woman, 1 week post vaginal delivery, with a tender abdomen, clean wound, pyrexia not responding to broad-spectrum antibiotics but subsequently responding to intravenous heparin.

4.69 A woman with a brisk vaginal bleed 2 weeks after a normal delivery.

THEME: URINARY INCONTINENCE

A Bladder cancer
B Detrusor overactivity
C Interstitial cystitis
D Overflow incontinence
E Urinary tract infection
F Urodynamic stress incontinence
G Vesicovaginal fistula

Instructions: From the list above choose the condition that matched the clinical pictures described below. Each option can be used once, more than once or not at all.

4.70 After an obstructed labour a woman had continuously leaking urine 3 weeks after delivery.

4.71 An obese patient complains of urgency and nocturia.

4.72 During urodynamic studies, a demonstrable leak on coughing is the only finding noted.

THEME: GYNAECOLOGICAL CANCER

A Endometrial cancer
B Cancer of the fallopian tube
C Cervical cancer
D Metastatic cancer
E Ovarian cancer
F Ovarian fibroma
G Vulval cancer

Instructions: On the basis of suspicion of which malignancy from the list above would the patient in the scenarios described below be urgently referred to hospital. Each option can be used once, more than once or not at all.

4.73 A 58-year-old woman presents with vaginal discharge and bleeding for 4 weeks. She is not taking any hormone replacement therapy.

4.74 A 30-year-old woman presents with post-coital bleeding and intermenstrual bleeding since 2 months.

4.75 A 75-year-old woman with a long-standing history of lichen sclerosus presents with swollen groin nodes since 3 months.

THEME: VULVAL DISEASE

A Corticosteroid cream
B Metronidazole gel
C Lidocaine gel
D Oestradiol cream for 2 weeks
E Silicone barrier cream
F Testosterone cream

Instructions: From the list above choose the most appropriate medication for the patients presenting to your general practice with the clinical pictures described below. Each option can be used once, more than once or not at all.

4.76 A 60-year-old woman with a clinical picture of atrophic vaginitis confirmed by histological examination.

4.77 A 35-year-old patient with severe urinary incontinence complaining of vulval irritation.

4.78 A 66-year-old woman with vulval soreness has had a vulval biopsy that has revealed lichen sclerosus.

THEME: THROMBOPROPHYLAXIS

A Anticoagulation (therapeutic) dose of low-molecular-weight heparin (LMWH) commenced post partum
B Anticoagulation (therapeutic) dose of LMWH given antenatally and post partum
C Prophylactic dose of LMWH commenced post partum
D Prophylactic dose of LMWH given antenatally and post partum
E Unfractionated heparin commenced post partum
F Unfractionated heparin given antenatally and post partum
G Warfarin given both antenatally and post partum

Instructions: From the list above choose the most appropriate treatment regimen for the conditions described below. Note that the duration of treatment is not specified. Each option can be used once, more than once or not at all.

4.79 A pregnant woman with a single deep vein thrombosis in the past. She has a normal thrombophilia screen and a negative family history.

4.80 A pregnant woman at her booking visit who is taking long-term warfarin for multiple thromboembolic events.

4.81 A healthy woman who has had an emergency caesarean section.

THEME: PRENATAL DIAGNOSTIC TESTING

A Amniocentesis at 7–9 weeks' gestation
B Amniocentesis at 11–13 weeks' gestation
C Amniocentesis at 15–18 weeks' gestation
D Chorionic villus sampling (CVS) at 7–9 weeks' gestation
E CVS at 11–13 weeks' gestation
F CVS at 15–18 weeks' gestation
G Testing not indicated

Instructions: From the list above choose the most appropriate advice to give to a woman who requests a diagnostic test for Down syndrome. Each option can be used once, more than once or not at all.

4.82 A pregnant woman with a previous baby affected by Down syndrome requests a diagnostic test to be performed as soon as it is safe to do so.

4.83 A woman wants to know which diagnostic test has the lowest risk to the fetus in order to plan a diagnostic test for Down syndrome.

4.84 A woman requests the safest test which can give a rapid result (within 48 hours) for Down syndrome. Which procedure is recommended?

THEME: MISCARRIAGE

A Ectopic pregnancy
B Missed miscarriage
C Molar pregnancy
D Recurrent miscarriage
E Septic miscarriage
F Spontaneous miscarriage
G Termination of pregnancy

Instructions: From the list above choose the option that matches the clinical presentations given below. Each option can be used once, more than once or not at all.

4.85 It affects approximately 10% of pregnancies and has a good prognosis for future pregnancies without intervention.

4.86 Ultrasound scan findings demonstrate there is no fetal heart and the scan has a snow storm appearance.

4.87 It affects 1% of couples and need further specialised investigations such as karyotyping.

THEME: MENSTRUAL ABNORMALITIES

A Fibroid uterus
B McCune–Albright syndrome
C Meigs syndrome
D Polycystic ovary syndrome
E Premenstrual syndrome
F Sheehan syndrome
G Turner syndrome
H Weight loss

Instructions: From the list above choose the single most likely cause for the conditions given below. Each option can be used once, more than once or not at all.

4.88 Hirsutism

4.89 Primary amenorrhoea

4.90 Precocious puberty

Practice Paper 4
Answers

BEST OF FIVE ANSWERS

4.1 A: Müllerian duct anomaly

Syphilis, antiphospholipid antibody, uterine and cervical anomalies can all cause recurrent second trimester miscarriages. Malaria and toxoplasmosis can cause sporadic miscarriage.

4.2 D: Cervical growth

If there is an obvious cervical growth, a cervical biopsy should be taken and examination under anaesthesia should be carried out. Colposcopy is also indicated in women with a suspicious looking cervix that bleeds on touch.

4.3 D: Increased risk of congenital malformation

Antiphospholipid antibody syndrome is related to large placental infarcts and venous thrombosis, and therefore placental insufficiency and IUGR. It can lead to first trimester and second trimester miscarriage and stillbirths.

4.4 B: It may lead in haematosalpinx and infertility

In imperforate hymen is usually diagnosed at puberty with cyclical pain and amenorrhoea. Treatment is incision. Müllerian duct malformations are associated with renal anomalies and not imperforate hymen. Vaginal reconstructive surgery is needed in cases of absent vagina.

Questions on pages 217–226

4.5 A: Check placenta and membranes for completeness

Retained fragments of placenta is a common cause for an atonic uterus. Placenta and membranes should be checked for completeness as first step. Simple measures such as B-Lynch sutures should be then be tried as internal iliac artery ligation needs special skills. Primary postpartum haemorrhage is mostly due to an atonic uterus while primary postpartum haemorrhage after 24 hours is due to endometritis or retained placental fragments.

4.6 E: Polycystic ovarian disease

This woman most likely has polycystic ovarian syndrome, which could be associated with hirsutism.

4.7 E: Cabergoline

Cabergoline is used for treatment of hyperprolactinaemia, and therefore best avoided when a woman wishes to breast feed.

4.8 B: Intravenous opiate misuse

IV opiate misuse is not a contraindication for epidural. Rather, pain control can be difficult in women taking iv drugs. Pethidine alone is probably not the best for pain control in iv drug misusers.

4.9 A: Hydrocephalus

Microcephaly is a feature of congenital rubella infection, hydrocephalus is not.

4.10 E: Early intubation + nasogastric tube

A baby with a diaphragmatic hernia needs early intubation and a nasogastric tube to prevent overdistension of stomach.

4.11 D: Maternal hyperthyroidism on treatment

Maternal hyperthyroidism if treated with propranolol could be a cause for bradycardia. Fetal tachycardia is a feature in presence of maternal infection and fetal prematurity.

4.12 C: Shoulder dystocia

Diabetes, obesity, postdate pregnancy and instrumental delivery are known risk factors for shoulder dystocia.

4.13 D: If performed at term may reduce the incidence of operative delivery

Should be performed at 36/37 weeks. When performed at 37 weeks it the incidence of operative delivery. Use of tocolysis may increase the rate of success but it does not reduce the rate of complications.

4.14 D: Stop insulin, glucose tolerance test 6 weeks later

Women with gestational diabetes do not need insulin after delivery, however a glucose tolerance test should be arranged at 6 weeks and the next pregnancy. They are also more likely to develop type 2 diabetes later in life therefore need regular checks.

4.15 D: Menopausal symptoms

Menopausal symptoms are not increased as oestrogen levels are higher in obese woman.

4.16 D: Undernutrition

Improved nutrition and increased body fat is associated with early menarche. McCune–Albright syndrome is characterised by café-au-lait spots, polyostotic fibrous dysplasia and precocious puberty.

4.17 D: Oestrogen + progesterone

Oestrogen gives relief from hot flushes but it should never be given alone in a woman with an intact uterus. Raloxifene and tibolone are not helpful in hot flushes.

4.18 D: Hypoparathyroidism

Hyperparathyroidism is related to secondary osteoporosis not hypoparathyroidism. All other given conditions can contribute to bone mineral loss.

4.19 C: Smoking

Smoking is inversely related to pregnancy-related hypertension. Primipara, positive family history and twin gestation all contribute towards her increased risk of pre-eclampsia.

4.20 E: Hyperemesis gravidarum

Hyperemesis is the most likely cause of such symptoms in pregnant women at 8 weeks of gestation; it can cause weight loss and epigastric pain secondary to heartburn. Other medical conditions should also be ruled out.

MULTIPLE CHOICE ANSWERS

4.21 BDE

In a menstruating woman if the COC is started on day 1 then extra precautions are not required for 7 days. If the COC is started on day 3 or later extra precautions are required for 7 days. If a woman is post partum and not lactating then the COC can be started on day 21 when there is a low risk of thrombosis. As first ovulation has been reported by day 28 extra precautions are not needed if started on day 21. During lactation COCs are not recommended. Progestogen-only injectables are preferred. After induced early abortion or miscarriage COCs can be started on the same or next day to avoid postoperative vomiting. Extra precautions are not needed for 7 days.

4.22 ACD

Cephalohaematoma is caused by bleeding that occurs below the periosteum and is associated with a ventouse delivery. Sometimes the swelling takes a long time to resolve and may actually lead to a calcified ridge. The resolution can be associated with an increased bilirubin level. Physiological jaundice occurs between days 2 and 5. Owing to the immaturity of the liver enzymes, there is a raised level of unconjugated bilirubin. Infection may lead to jaundice and it is therefore important to investigate these babies. Full blood count, blood cultures, lumbar puncture, chest X-ray and midstream urine specimen are important investigations. If rhesus incompatibility is suspected, investigations should include:

- Coombs test
- maternal blood group
- infant blood group

... cont

Questions on pages 227–242

- Detection of anti-A or anti-B haemolysins in the maternal circulation.

Hypothyroidism is associated with jaundice, but this is a prolonged jaundice.

4.23 C

The dangers of hypoxia and fetal trauma are greater in the flexed/footling types. Meconium often reflects pressure on the fetal abdomen and is not a reliable sign of distress. Variable fetal heart rate decelerations are commonly due to cord compression. Elective caesarean section, in many units, is the preferred mode of delivery. Obstetric forceps allow safe delivery of the aftercoming head by ensuring the head is not delivered too slowly, which can result in cerebral hypoxia, nor too rapidly, which may cause intracranial haemorrhage.

4.24 ABC

It is important to know the common side-effects of drugs. Oestrogen is often associated with weight gain, although studies have not always confirmed this. Aciclovir, which is the treatment for herpes simplex and varicella zoster, can cause a rash and gastrointestinal disturbances as well as rise in bilirubin and liver enzymes. It can also cause increased levels of blood urea and creatinine, headache, fatigue and neurological reactions such as dizziness. Fluconazole, used in the treatment of thrush, can cause nausea, abdominal discomfort, diarrhoea and flatulence and occasionally it can also cause abnormalities of the liver enzymes. Bromocriptine can cause nausea, vomiting, constipation, headaches, dizziness and postural hypotension. In particular, vasospasm in fingers can occur in patients with Raynaud syndrome. Danazol has an androgenic effect and is therefore associated with reduction in breast size as well as acne, oily skin and possible hirsutism.

4.25 BCE

Obesity is a risk factor for hypertension but not for pre-eclampsia. Women who have had hypertension while taking a combined oral contraceptive are at risk, as are those with autoimmune disorders.

4.26 BC

Increasing maternal age increases the incidence of a hydatidiform mole. Surgical evacuation with human chorionic gonadotrophin follow-up is the treatment of choice. Choriocarcinoma is treated by methotrexate and other chemotherapeutic agents.

4.27 ABE

The signs and symptoms of ovarian cancer have been described as vague or silent; about 10% of ovarian cancer is diagnosed in the early stages. Symptoms typically occur in advanced stages and may include any of the following: loss of appetite, nausea and a bloated feeling, unexplained weight gain, abdominal distension, abnormal vaginal bleeding, and changes in bowel or bladder habits. Most of the ovarian tumours are of epithelial origin, and these are rare before the age of 35 years. The incidence increases with age and peaks in the 50–70-year age group. CA125 is a tumour marker for ovarian cancer. About half the women who have early-stage ovarian cancer do not have raised levels of CA125. Also, it can be raised in a variety of other conditions, such as endometriosis, fibroids, pelvic inflammatory disease, and even pregnancy.

4.28 ACD

There were 155 deaths were due to indirect causes and 106 were due to direct causes in 2000–2002. In 1997–1999 there were 136 deaths due to indirect causes and 106 deaths due to direct causes. Deaths due to hypertensive disease remain unchanged. There was also a rise in deaths due to anaesthesia-related causes. Thromboembolism as the most common cause of direct deaths remained unchanged.

4.29 BCDE

The highest incidence of damage is 50% at 4 weeks. The risk decreases after the first trimester. Gammaglobulin, if given, may be protective.

4.30 ABCE

Uterovaginal prolapse results from weakness of the pelvic support, including muscles, ligaments and fascia. Multiparity, long labour, instrumental deliveries and vaginal delivery of large babies are some of the factors that predispose a woman to developing uterine prolapse. The menopause can weaken the pelvic floor because of diminished oestrogen levels. Increased intra-abdominal pressure on a long-term basis can contribute to genital prolapse, for example, heavy lifting, obesity, ascites and chronic coughing and chronic constipation are important contributing factors in genital prolapse. No relation has been found between uterovaginal prolapse and LLETZ.

4.31 AE

Endometrial carcinoma tends to spread to lymphatics in the later stages or when there is extensive myometrial invasion. Radiotherapy is contraindicated in the presence of sepsis. A Wertheim hysterectomy entails the excision of uterus, tubes, often ovaries, upper third of the vagina, parametria and pelvic lymph nodes. The ovaries are excised in cases of carcinoma of the endometrium, as they are a site for malignant spread or oestrogen production, and the disease usually occurs in the postmenopausal age group. Renal failure usually occurs in carcinoma of the cervix due to the tumour obstructing both ureters.

4.32 ABDE

Rubella, an RNA virus spread by droplet infection, is associated with a mild viral illness with macular papular rash and lymphadenopathy. Over 90% of women in the UK who attend antenatal clinics are immune to rubella. Toxoplasmosis is due to a protozoan, *Toxoplasma gondii*, and the oocysts are found in raw meat and cat faeces. It is a rare congenital infection occurring in approximately 1:100 000 births. Congenital infection occurs in 30% of infants whose mothers sero-convert during pregnancy and this can lead to stillbirth, neonatal death or severe handicap. The treatment of choice is spiramycin. Varicella is a febrile illness in the mother, with a characteristic rash, a relation of the virus known as shingles. The congenital varicella syndrome, which is associated with skin scarring, is rare. *Listeria* is a Gram-positive bacillus associated with a non-specific febrile illness in the mother. It is specifically found in soft cheeses and prepacked food and infection occurs in approximately 1:700 pregnancies. It is associated with spontaneous miscarriage, stillbirth and neonatal death, and the infection can be treated with ampicillin.

4.33 ABDE

D&C was the classical method of obtaining samples of the endometrium, having first been reported in 1843. In 1989–1990 it was one of the most common procedures performed, although it is increasingly being replaced by outpatient procedures as well as the use of the hysteroscope. A D&C does not sample all the endometrium and it has been shown that up to 5% of lesions are missed, including polyps, hyperplasia and even carcinoma. A D&C is not without risks and these include cervical tears, haemorrhage and even death following uterine perforation and damage to the bowel.

4.34 ABCDE

In uncomplicated vulvovaginal candidiasis topical antifungals will achieve clinical cure in 80% of cases. Oral azoles are contraindicated in pregnancy. Topical creams should also be used in conjunction with vaginal pessaries such as clotrimazole, econazole and miconazole.

4.35 BCD

The rise in progesterone during pregnancy can cause a decrease in gut motility and thus constipation. Iron therapy can aggravate the problem.

4.36 BD

During pregnancy, fasting plasma glucose concentration is decreased, probably due to the haemodilution effect of the increased plasma volume. The glomerular filtration rate is increased in normal pregnancy; this may lead to the renal threshold being exceeded and to glycosuria without impaired glucose tolerance. Fasting plasma insulin concentration rises in late pregnancy to accompany the increased glucose requirements. Glucose tolerance alters during pregnancy; although plasma glucose levels should have returned to normal 2 hours after an oral glucose load, insulin concentration often remains raised.

4.37 BCE

Androgen insensitivity syndrome is associated with chromosomal pattern of 46XY. Usually polycystic ovarian disease presents late, but it could be a possibility in this case. In primary ovarian failure there would be higher levels of the luteinising and follicle-stimulating hormones. Imperforate hymen may be an option and the patient may also complain of cyclical pain and abdominal swelling.

4.38 CD

The organisms commonly responsible for meningitis in children and adults are relatively uncommon as a cause among newborns.

4.39 BDE

The death rate was 13/100 000. There was increase in deaths due to anaesthesia.

4.40 ABCE

The copper intrauterine device can cause increased menstrual blood loss, irregular bleeding and increased period pain.

4.41 CDE

Dietary advice should focus on a well-balanced and varied diet with adequate daily folate, iron, calcium (1200 mg) and fluids (2–3 litres). Foods likely to have *Listeria* should be avoided, eg raw meat, raw seafood and soft cheeses. Exercise is commonly restricted to non-contact sports after 16 weeks. Ideally, vigorous exercise should be limited to 15–20 minutes. There are good data to show that pelvic floor exercise undertaken antenatally results in stronger pelvic floor muscles postnatally, and this may have an influence on continence status and genital prolapse in the future. Problems may arise at different times during pregnancy, so the assessment for risk factors and complications must be an ongoing process throughout pregnancy, labour, delivery and in the postpartum period. Some women will require more visits than others. A minimum of four antenatal visits is recommended for a woman with a normal pregnancy (Antenatal Care Report of a Technical Working Group. Geneva: World Health Organization, 1994).

4.42 BD

Pruritus vulva is the term used to describe itching affecting the genital area of women. It should be distinguished from vulvodynia, which refers to chronic burning symptoms. Skin conditions such as dermatitis, psoriasis and lichen sclerosus can cause pruritus vulvae. At least 10% of women all over the world have this problem. One of the main causes of pruritus vulvae is purulent and mucopurulent vaginal discharge and it is seen in over 80% of cases. Glycosuria and diabetes also contribute to this condition.

4.43 ACE

The International Society for the Study of Vulvovaginal Disease (ISSVD) defines vulvodynia as chronic vulval discomfort or pain. It is characterised by itching, burning or a stinging or stabbing pain in a vulva in which there is no infection or skin disease of the vulva or vagina. The pain can be unprovoked, varying from constant to intermittent. It is also known as vulvar vestibulitis syndrome or vestibulodynia. Often the vagina shows no abnormalities or signs of infection. Unfortunately, many doctors are unaware of this condition and may suggest to their patients that it is a psychological condition.

4.44 AB

For an uncomplicated pregnancy, labour can be induced with vaginal prostaglandin agents on the antenatal ward. However, in women with recognised risk factors (including suspected fetal growth retardation or previous caesarean section) induction should not occur on an antenatal ward. Wherever labour is induced, facilities should be available for continuous fetal heart rate monitoring. Cardiotocography should be established immediately prior to induction of labour. Prolonged use of maternal facial oxygen treatment may be harmful to the fetus and should be avoided. Where oxytocin is being used for induction or augmentation of labour, continuous electronic fetal monitoring should be used.

4.45 CDE

Physical signs suggestive of early pregnancy include changes in the breasts and the Hegar sign, a softening of the cervical isthmus, occurring around 6 weeks' gestation. Physical signs during the first trimester are unreliable predictors of pregnancy (low sensitivity). The average duration of pregnancy is 266 days from the date of ovulation. If calculation is made according to the first day of the last menstrual period, the average duration is 280 days. Ovulation most frequently occurs on the 14th day of a 28-day cycle. The uterus begins to enlarge shortly after implantation and 4 weeks after conception, the rate of enlargement is approximately 1 cm per week. Fifty per cent of pregnant women will experience nausea and vomiting between 2 weeks and 12 weeks after conception.

4.46 CD

Fertilisation of the human ovum occurs in the lateral or ampullary part of the uterine tube approximately 12–24 hours after ovulation, and the ovum then passes along the tube to the cavity of the uterus where implantation occurs approximately 5–7 days after fertilisation. Fertilisation comprises the union of the spermatozoon with the mature ovum. Under normal conditions only one spermatozoon enters the ovum and takes part in the process of fertilisation. Spermatogenesis occurs in the seminiferous tubules of the testes and begins at puberty.

4.47 ABE

Trophoblastic cells produce hCG. Serum levels of this hormone rise steadily during the first 6 weeks of pregnancy. During this early stage of pregnancy, hCG levels double every 1.3–2 days. Modern urine pregnancy tests can detect hCG concentrations as low as 25 mIU/ml; 98% of women will have positive urinary pregnancy test by 7 days after implantation. Radioimmunoassay techniques for measuring concentrations of serum P-hCG can detect levels as low as 2–10 mIU/ml.

4.48 ABCDE

The following are all risk factors for ectopic pregnancy:

- Previous history of pelvic inflammatory disease or other pelvic infection. *Chlamydia* and *Gonorrhoea* can both grow within the fallopian tubes and cause damage to the endosalpinx and peritubal adhesions. Other pelvic infections, such as appendicitis, can also result in pelvic adhesions and thus increase the chances of an ectopic pregnancy.
- Previous tubal surgery, such as reversed sterilisation with tubal reanastomosis, microsurgery for infertility and unexpected pregnancy after sterilisation.
- Previous ectopic pregnancy. There is a roughly 10-fold increase in ectopic pregnancy.
- Intrauterine contraceptive device (IUCD) in situ. All but the progesterone-containing IUCDs are relatively protective against ectopic pregnancy while the IUCD is in place. That is, the number of ectopic pregnancies in women using an IUCD for contraception is about half that in women using no contraception. However, when IUCD pregnancies occur there is a greater chance of an ectopic location (3–4%).
- Assisted conception technology (in vitro fertilisation and gamete intrafallopian transfer). The risk of a heterotopic pregnancy (previously thought to be 1 per 30 000 pregnancies) increased markedly in women conceiving with one of the assisted reproductive technologies (up to 1 per 100 pregnancies).
- A history of diethylstilboestrol exposure in utero. There are often uterine cavity defects that may limit intrauterine implantation. Also, tubal defects exist that may increase the chance for a tubal ectopic pregnancy.

4.49 ABCE

hCG is detectable in the blood or urine 1–2 days after implantation (10 days after ovulation). It increases rapidly (doubling every 36–48 hours in the first six weeks), reaching a peak 60–80 days after fertilisation; then drops off quickly to 10–30% of the peak value for the rest of the pregnancy. It serves to maintain progesterone production by the corpus luteum in the early part of pregnancy, and also stimulates the development of the fetal gonads and synthesis of androgens. At levels of 1000–1500 IU/l, an intrauterine sac should normally be seen using transvaginal ultrasound.

4.50 ABCDE

The incidence of cord prolapse is 0.14–0.62% with a perinatal mortality between 8.6% and 49%. There are several recognised risk factors including:

- Abnormal presentation (breech, transverse lie and oblique lie)
- High parity
- High presenting part
- Multiple pregnancy
- Pelvic tumours
- Preterm rupture of membranes
- Polyhydramnios

4.51 CD

Screening is now recommended from 25 years of age, performed 3 yearly until 50 years then 5 yearly. Moderate and severe dyskaryosis, persistent borderline nuclear abnormalities, glandular changes, two successive mild dyskaryosis and suspected cancer are indications for referral for colposcopy.

4.52 BE

Primary amenorrhoea is defined as absence of menstruation at 16 years of age when secondary sexual characteristics are present and 14 years in their absence. Chromosomal analysis is important to diagnose mosaicism (ovotestis) as surgical removal of the gonad is important in such cases as these patients have high risk of malignancy. Treatment for testicular feminisation is removal of testis. Biopsy is not always warranted as a diagnosis can be reached by raised gonadotrophin levels.

4.53 AB

Tubal factors are the commonest cause of female infertility. PCOS is the commonest cause for anovulation. Thirty per cent of unexplained infertility patients conceive in 3 years of conservative treatment. Routine hysteroscopy is not recommended by the Royal College of Obstetricians and Gynaecologists.

4.54 ABC

Maternal age and uterine surgery are risk factors for placenta praevia.

4.55 BDE

Uterine rupture is less common with elective repeat caesarean. Risk of perineal injury is reduced with elective caesarean section.

4.56 BCD

Heart rate, breathing, reflex, colour and tone are used for Apgar scoring. Blood pressure and meconium are not used.

4.57 D

All of the others can cause postpartum collapse.

4.58 ABCE

Racial differences are shown is some studies with higher incidence in Caucasians, however, it might only reflect cultural differences in reporting.

4.59 ABC

Arousal problems, essential vulvodynia and episiotomy could be causative factors for dyspareunia.

4.60 ABCE

Treatment of partners is ineffective. Pregnant women should be treated with topical anti-fungal agents.

EXTENDING MATCHING ANSWERS

THEME: MATERNAL MORTALITY

4.61 I Thromboembolism.

4.62 D Cardiac disease.

4.63 H Psychiatric causes. For the categories of direct and indirect deaths, deaths up to 42 days after delivery are included. If deaths up to 1 year are included psychiatric causes become more common, particularly deaths from suicide.

THEME: VAGINAL BIRTH AFTER CAESAREAN SECTION

4.64 D Previous classic caesarean section. The risk of rupture in a trial of vaginal delivery is 2–9% when a classic caesarean has been performed in a previous pregnancy.

4.65 B Elective repeat caesarean section. There is virtually no risk of a uterine rupture in a woman undergoing an elective repeat caesarean section.

4.66 E Previous vaginal delivery, especially a successful birth after caesarean section, is the best predictor of a successful birth after caesarean section.

Questions on pages 243–252

THEME: POSTNATAL PROBLEMS

4.67 G Typical features of a urinary tract infection. The picture could be similar with endometritis but the lochia would usually be offensive in endometritis.

4.68 F Septic pelvic thrombophlebitis. The diagnosis is often difficult. The response to antibiotics and heparin is typical.

4.69 C Endometritis. A secondary postpartum bleed is often due to endometritis with or without retained products of conception.

THEME: URINARY INCONTINENCE

4.70 G Vesicovaginal fistula presents with continuously leaking urine.

4.71 B Detrusor overactivity. Urgency and nocturia are clinical features of detrusor overactivity.

4.72 F Urodynamic stress incontinence. A demonstrable leak is taken as diagnostic.

THEME: GYNAECOLOGICAL CANCER

4.73 A Endometrial cancer. Any postmenopausal vaginal discharge or bleeding must be taken as caused by endometrial cancer until proven otherwise. Urgent endometrial sampling must be undertaken.

4.74 C Cervical cancer. This classically presents with post-coital bleeding that much be investigated urgently.

4.75 G Vulval cancer. Women with lichen sclerosus need regular life-long follow up with vulval biopsies whenever suspicious areas are found. This is because there is a 3% risk of developing vulval cancer.

THEME: VULVAL DISEASE

4.76 D Oestradiol cream for 2 weeks. A short, low-dose dermal course of oestradiol would not increase the risk of endometrial cancer and would help with atrophic vaginitis.

4.77 E Silicone barrier cream. Urine leakage causes ammoniacal dermatitis and excoriation, and the liberal use of this cream should be encouraged.

4.78 A Corticosteroid cream. A potent corticosteroid cream will control symptoms.

THEME: THROMBOPROPHYLAXIS

4.79 C The major period of risk is post partum therefore prophylactic LMWH treatment should begin after delivery.

4.80 B Warfarin should be discontinued in favour of anticoagulant (therapeutic) doses of LMWH in the antenatal period. Approximately 1 week after delivery when the risk of bleeding is reduced warfarin can be re-started. LMWH should be given until satisfactory anticoagulation is achieved with warfarin.

4.81 C LMWH is given prophylactically until fully mobile.

THEME: PRENATAL DIAGNOSTIC TESTING

4.82 E CVS at 11–13 weeks' gestation. CVS is not performed in most units before 10 weeks' gestation because of the risks of a possible association with limb reduction defects. CVS is safer than amniocentesis before 14 weeks.

4.83 C Amniocentesis at 15–18 weeks' gestation. The rate of miscarriage associated with amniocentesis is approximately 1%. CVS is associated with a higher rate of miscarriage than second trimester amniocentesis.

4.84 C Amniocentesis at 15–18 weeks' gestation. New techniques for the provision of results by QF-PCR (quantitative florescent polymerase chain reaction) or FISH (fluorescent in situ hybridisation) can give rapid results using specimens obtained via amniocentesis.

THEME: MISCARRIAGE

4.85 F Spontaneous miscarriage.

4.86 C Molar pregnancy.

4.87 D Recurrent miscarriage.

THEME: MENSTRUAL ABNORMALITIES

4.88 D Polycystic ovary syndrome. Typically there is hirsutism, oligomenorrhoea and subfertility.

4.89 G Turner syndrome.

4.90 B McCune–Albright syndrome presents with precocious puberty and cystic bone changes.

Practice Paper 5 Questions

BEST OF FIVE QUESTIONS

20 Questions: Time allowed 30 minutes. Please give the single most appropriate answer from the list of alternatives.

5.1 Which one of the medications listed below can be prescribed to a woman taking an oral contraceptive without affecting the efficacy of her contraception or the therapeutic effect of the medication itself?

- A Insulin
- B Barbiturates
- C Rifampicin
- D Griseofulvin
- E Phenytoin

5.2 An unbooked patient with no previous scans presents at an estimated 43 weeks' gestation. Which one of the following is most unlikely to be the cause for her postmature pregnancy?

- A Fetal adrenal hypoplasia
- B Extrauterine pregnancy
- C Wrong dates
- D Placental sulphatase deficiency
- E Maternal diabetes

Answers on pages 317–320

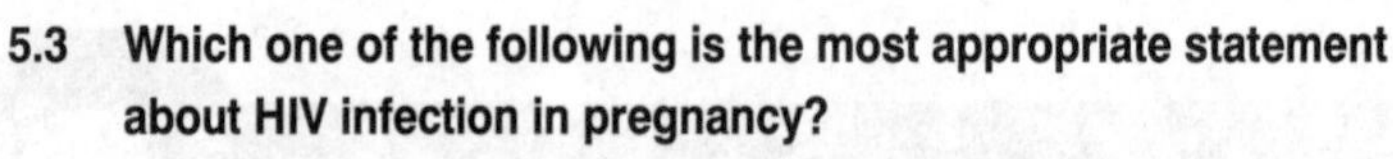

5.3 Which one of the following is the most appropriate statement about HIV infection in pregnancy?

- A Incidence of pre-eclampsia is higher in HIV+ patients
- B Vaginal delivery is absolutely contraindicated
- C Instrumental delivery is contraindicated
- D Breast feeding is not contraindicated
- E Pregnancy does not accelerate the course of HIV

5.4 A para 2 has delivered a 4.8 kg baby. She had shoulder dystocia during this delivery. Which one of the following is not likely to be the cause for the big baby?

- A Maternal obesity
- B Maternal toxoplasmosis
- C Previous macrosomic baby
- D Post-term pregnancy
- E Maternal diabetes

5.5 A low-risk para 1 is in labour at 4 cm on admission to labour ward. A student midwife accidently performed an amniotomy while examining her. Which one of the following is the most likely result from this accident?

- A Reduction in labour duration by 60–120 min
- B Decrease in the risk of caesarean delivery
- C A better 5 min Apgar score
- D An increase in the use of oxytocin
- E Increased risk of admission to the neonatal intensive care unit

5.6 Different maternal and fetal factors can contribute to cephalopelvic disproportion. Which one of the following conditions in a pregnant woman is most likely to contribute to achieve a normal vaginal delivery?

- A Severe kyphoscoliosis
- B Pelvic kidney
- C Hydrocephalus
- D Brow presentation
- E Face presentation – mento-anterior position

5.7 You are called to attend delivery of a pregnant woman with meconium in the second stage of labour. Which one of the following you are most likely to avoid while dealing with the newborn?

- A Clearing mouth and nose of secretions
- B Dry and stimulate the baby
- C Give oxygen as necessary
- D Routine endotracheal suctioning to clear the trachea of meconium
- E Mechanical respiration as necessary

5.8 You are assisting an specialist registrar with an instrumental delivery. The woman was delivered by forceps in lithotomy position and had an episiotomy and a vaginal tear. Which one of the following is the most appropriate statement about perineal trauma in such cases?

A Instrumental delivery increases risk of perineal trauma, and approximately 10% women experience ultrasound visible anal sphincter defect

B Episiotomy reduces posterior vaginal wall trauma

C Episiotomy is recommended for instrumental delivery based on evidence

D Delivery in the lithotomy position reduces the chance of perineal trauma

E Rectal examination is not recommended while repairing perineal tears

5.9 The mother of a newborn is worried about her baby. A number of situations are normal and some will need further investigation and treatment. In which one of the following situations will the neonate need to be investigated/treated further?

A A neonate who has not passed urine in 12 hours should be investigated for renal or obstructive cause

B A breast-fed infant loses weight in the first week of life

C Rectal temperature < 36 °C

D Erythema toxicum

E Cephalhaematoma

5.10 You are counselling a woman who has been recently diagnosed as having polycystic ovarian syndrome (PCOS) about long-term risks associated with the disease. Which one of the following has the least chance of happening?

- A Increased incidence of type 2 diabetes
- B Increased risk of gestational diabetes
- C Increased risk of pregnancy-induced hypertension
- D Marked increase in mortality from circulatory disease
- E Endometrial hyperplasia

5.11 Progesterone-only contraception is unlikely to act through which one of these mechanisms?

- A Thickens cervical mucus and inhibits sperm penetration
- B Endometrial modification to prevent implantation
- C Affects fallopian tube motility and therefore impairs sperm migration and ovum transport
- D Local effect on ovary and suppresses follicular growth and inhibits luteal activity
- E Inhibits ovulation by inhibiting by cyclical release of follicle-stimulating hormone and luteinising hormone

5.12 A para 2 woman is requesting insertion of an intrauterine contraceptive device (IUCD). In the presence of which one of the following conditions is it acceptable practice to perform an IUCD insertion on her request.

A Menorrhagia and anaemia

B Undiagnosed vaginal bleeding

C Active or recent pelvic inflammatory disease (within the past 3 months)

D Distorted uterine cavity

E Suspected malignancy of the genitalia

5.13 A 1.9 m (6 feet 8 inches) tall man with gynaecomastia, small testes and oligozoospermia presents at your clinic. Which one of the following is the most likely chromosomal karyotype of this man?

A 46,XXY

B 46,XO

C 46,XY

D 46,XYY

E 45,XXY

5.14 A woman was treated with danazol for endometriosis and has developed signs of virilisation. Danazol is discontinued. Which one of her symptoms is most likely to persist?

- A Breast atrophy
- B Male-type baldness
- C Deepening of voice
- D Hirsutism and oily skin
- E Weight gain

5.15 Prenatal diagnosis of which one the following conditions is specifically important in a male fetus only?

- A Tay–Sach disease
- B β-Thalassaemia
- C Cystic fibrosis
- D Congenital adrenal hyperplasia
- E Duchenne muscular dystrophy

5.16 Which one of the following is the most appropriate statement regarding ultrasound, when it is used to detect fetal abnormalities?

- A It has high specificity with variable sensitivity
- B Neural tube defects are missed in 40% of cases
- C Calyceal dilatation if present due to any cause is detected at the 20-week anatomical scan
- D Cardiac abnormalities can be easily detected
- E Abnormalities are detected better when performed after 20 weeks

5.17 With regards to analgesics and anaesthesia during labour. Which one of the following is the most accurate statement?

A Epidural anaesthesia prolongs the duration of first stage of labour

B Transmission of pain in first stage of labour is related to T10–T12 and L1 level

C Transmission of pain in the second stage of labour is related to L2–L5 spinal level

D Epidural anaesthesia causes hypertension

E Spinal anaesthesia is better than epidural with regard to blood pressure control

5.18 A 48-year-old woman presents with a pelvic mass 10 cm in size. Ultrasound shows a complex ovarian cyst on the left ovary with papillary growth and multiloculation. The CA125 level is 250 I. u/l. Which one of the following is most appropriate management plan for her?

A Laparotomy and biopsy to confirm malignancy

B Left oophorectomy

C Abdominal hysterectomy and left oophorectomy

D Chemotherapy

E Referral to a gynaecological oncologist

5.19 A 7-week pregnant gravida 3 with history of two miscarriages who smokes 10 cigarettes/day presents with hyperemesis gravidarum. Which one of the following would be most appropriate statement when counselling her?

- A The incidence is high in smokers
- B Ginger can be used for treatment
- C More common in pregnancy associated with hypothyroidism
- D Seen more commonly in unsuccessful pregnancies
- E Is more frequent in older women

5.20 A primigravida at 35 weeks' gestation complaints of vaginal leakage. Which one of the following is most likely to be the next step in her management?

- A Induction of labour should be planned within the next 72 hours
- B Accurate diagnosis should be made by history and speculum examination
- C Digital vaginal examination should be performed to rule-out labour
- D Prescribe erythromycin to reduce maternal mortality
- E Prescribe co-amoxiclav to reduce neonatal complications

MULTIPLE CHOICE QUESTIONS

40 Questions: Time allowed 1½ hours. Indicate your answers clearly by putting a tick against the correct or true options and a cross against the incorrect or false options. (The section on answers in this book lists the correct (true) options.)

5.21 The following factors positively influence high birth weight:

A Maternal growth hormone

B Prolonged pregnancy (> 294 days)

C Fetal hyperinsulinaemia

D Primiparity

E Social class

5.22 Possible causes of an unstable lie include:

A Polyhydramnios

B Prematurity

C Uterine abnormality

D Placenta praevia

E Fibroid uterus

Answers on pages 321–334

5.23 A hysterosalpingogram:

A Confirms tubal function

B Can be used to diagnose uterine adhesions

C Is a diagnostic test for ectopic pregnancy

D When performed, should be accompanied by a prophylactic antibiotic

E Is useful in the assessment of the effect of fibroids in infertility

5.24 Bilateral salpingo-oophorectomy at the time of hysterectomy:

A Eliminates premenstrual syndrome

B Is technically more difficult than a hysterectomy

C Should never be performed in women under the age of 35

D Is the treatment of choice in stage 1 endometrial carcinoma

E Always requires postoperative hormone replacement therapy

5.25 Which of the following statements about vulvovaginal candidiasis is/are true?

A Thrush affects about 25% of women at least once in their life time

B *Candida albicans* is a commensal in the human genital and digestive tracts

C *Candida glabrata* causes 75–80% of vulvovaginal candidiasis

D Bubble bath causes vaginal thrush

E A raised pH of the vagina is diagnostic

5.26 Dysmenorrhoea:

A Is called primary if it occurs with ovulation

B If it is primary, is associated with an abnormal level of prostaglandins

C Is called secondary when an organic cause is found

D If secondary, may be caused by pelvic inflammatory disease

E If primary, the contraceptive pill is useful treatment

5.27 Which of the following statements about twin pregnancy is/are true?

A Monozygotic twins occur at a fairly constant rate

B It is associated with an increased risk of placenta praevia

C Reducing the number of embryos replaced during in vitro fertilisation (IVF) reduces the twinning risk

D The risk of dizygotic twins decreases with increasing maternal age and parity

E It is associated with an increased risk of gestational diabetes

5.28 Tubal patency is required for the following methods of assisted conception:

A Intrauterine insemination

B In vitro fertilisation

C Donor insemination

D Gamete intrafallopian transfer

E Ovum donation

5.29 Intrauterine contraceptive devices:

A Lead to an increase in the number of leukocytes in the endometrium and tubal fluid

B Cause a decrease in local prostaglandins

C Containing copper are toxic to sperm and the blastocyst

D Can contain a slow-release progestogen

E Are usually inert

5.30 The volume of amniotic fluid:

A Is independent of fetal urine production

B May be accurately measured by ultrasound

C Is excessive in severe rhesus disease

D Increases following amniocentesis

E Is reduced in severe pre-eclampsia

5.31 Heartburn in pregnancy:

A Affects about two-thirds of all women at some stage during pregnancy

B Is commonly associated with eating or lying down

C Can be treated effectively with diazepam

D Magnesium salts would appear to be one of the safest treatment options

E May be treated with dilute hydrochloric acid

5.32 Fetal biophysical profile scoring:

- A Has resulted in the birth of babies with lower Apgar scores
- B Has resulted in a reduction in the perinatal mortality rate
- C Includes serum oestradiol measurement
- D Includes fetal tone measurement on ultrasound scan
- E Includes fetal breathing assessment

5.33 Which of the following conditions is/are thought to be commonly caused by viruses?

- A Condyloma acuminatum
- B Bartholinitis
- C Cervical intraepithelial neoplasia
- D Lichen sclerosus
- E Acute vulval ulcers

5.34 Cervical cancer:

- A Human papillomavirus infection is a major risk factor for development of preinvasive or invasive carcinoma of the cervix
- B Cervical cancer can be presented as postmenopausal bleeding
- C The incidence of cervical carcinoma is 9.3 cases per 10 000 women
- D The UK has the highest recorded incidence in the European Union
- E Deaths from cervical cancer have fallen by more than 40%

5.35 A low haemoglobin in pregnancy:

- A Should initially be treated with iron
- B Depends on a complex relation between red cell mass and plasma volume
- C Is usually associated with an iron-deficiency anaemia
- D Can be improved more quickly with the addition of ascorbic acid
- E If associated with a megaloblastic anaemia in pregnancy, is almost always due to folate deficiency

5.36 Treatment of benign hirsutism includes:

- A The contraceptive pill
- B Danazol
- C Cyproterone acetate
- D Prednisolone
- E Electrolysis

5.37 Which of the following statements about perimenopausal contraception is/are true?

- A Measurement of the oestradiol levels is a valid method of identifying the menopause
- B It is accepted that contraception is required for a another 1 year when the menopause occurs in women over the age of 50 years
- C It is accepted that contraception is required for another 2 years when the menopause occurs in women under the age of 50 years
- D Hormone replacement therapy with progestogens is a reliable form of contraceptive
- E Follicle-stimulating hormone levels are reliable in women taking the progestogen-only pill as this does not affect testing

5.38 Vulval carcinoma:

- A Is associated with pruritus vulvae
- B Is usually multifocal
- C Is uncommon in African patients
- D Is more common in multiparous patients
- E Is best treated by chemotherapy

5.39 Polyhydramnios may be associated with:

- A Placental abruption
- B Intrauterine growth restriction
- C Fetal oesophageal atresia
- D Preterm labour
- E Postpartum haemorrhage

5.40 A progestogen:

- A Causes a withdrawal bleed on an oestrogen-primed endometrium
- B Can be used as a screening test for endometrial hyperplasia
- C Is the treatment of choice for menorrhagia
- D When given to a postmenopausal woman can cause a decrease in the incidence of endometrial carcinoma
- E Should be given routinely to all postmenopausal women who are on oestrogen treatment

5.41 With regard to breech presentation:

- A Incidence at term is 3%
- B Nulliparity and old age are associated factors
- C Elective caesarean section is performed at 38 weeks
- D External cephalic version should be offered at 37 weeks
- E Perinatal mortality/morbidity is highest in complete breech

5.42 With regard to urinary tract infection in pregnancy:

A Asymptomatic bacteriuria affects 5–7% of women

B It is recurrent in 30% of cases

C Acute pyelonephritis treatment should be continued for 7 days

D 20% cases of pyelonephritis can have underlying renal tract abnormality, therefore ultrasound is recommended

E Sulphonamides are the drug of choice

5.43 Which of the following statements about prolactinomas in pregnancy is/are true?

A Treatment with a dopamine receptor agonist should be stopped once pregnancy is confirmed

B 33% become symptomatic in pregnancy

C Risk of tumour expansion is maximum in third trimester

D Breast feeding is contraindicated

E Diagnosis is based on prolactin levels A

5.44 With regard to human immunodeficiency virus (HIV) infection in pregnancy:

A Management is by multidisciplinary team

B Baseline serology for cytomegalovirus and toxoplasmosis is checked at booking

C Vertical transmission rate without intervention is 15–30%

D Selective screening is offered to the high-risk population only

E Breast feeding is advised

5.45 Which of the following statements is/are true about vaccination in pregnancy?

A Rubella vaccination should be given in the second trimester

B At-risk women should be offered hepatitis B vaccine

C Tetanus toxoid is safe in pregnancy

D Postexposure prophylaxis is safe during pregnancy

E Cholera vaccination prevents spread of disease

5.46 Complications of amniocentesis include:

A Miscarriage

B Respiratory distress

C Limb reduction deformity if performed early

D Intrauterine growth restriction

E Feto-maternal haemorrhage

5.47 Methods of cervical priming include:

A Intravaginal prostraglandin (PG) E_2 gel

B Intracervical PGE_2 gel

C Misoprostol

D Intramuscular carboprost

E Intramuscular ergometrine

5.48 Risks and complications associated with induction of labour include:

- A Uterine hypostimulation
- B Neonatal jaundice
- C Water intoxication
- D Fetal distress
- E Prolonged second stage

5.49 Which of the following is/are true about a normal antenatal cardiotocograph?

- A Normal baseline is 100–160 beats/min
- B Beat to beat variability should be > 5 beats
- C Interpretation may be difficult prior to 32 weeks
- D There should be at least three accelerations in 20 minutes
- E It has high long-term prognostic value

5.50 Which of the following is/are true about labour?

- A In low-risk patients auscultation every 15 minutes should be done in first stage
- B Vaginal examination is done every 2 hours in low-risk primipara
- C Third stage should be actively managed by prostaglandins
- D Admission cardiotocography is mandatory for all women coming in labour
- E Women in labour with a previous caesarean should be continuously monitored

5.51 Which of the following statements about low-dose aspirin and pregnancy is/are true?

- A The usual dose is 75 mg/day
- B It is associated with an increased risk of accidental haemorrhage
- C It is useful in preventing the deterioration of pre-eclampsia
- D It may be useful in the prevention of recurrent miscarriage
- E It may be useful in thromboprophylaxis

5.52 *Gardnerella vaginalis*:

- A Is a Gram-negative bacillus
- B Is associated with clue cells, which are bacteria attached to vaginal epithelial cells
- C Is associated with a vaginal pH > 5
- D Can be transported on Stuart's medium
- E Generates a strawberry odour

5.53 Important guidelines for the management of recurrent vulvovaginal candidiasis include:

- A Symptoms of thrush are typically worse before and better after menstruation
- B Advice regarding avoidance of tightly fitting synthetic garments should be given
- C Treatment regimens that work well in cases of uncomplicated thrush may be ineffective in recurrent thrush
- D Clotrimazole 500 mg vaginally weekly is a useful maintenance therapy
- E Maintenance treatment should be given for no longer than a month

5.54 Ultrasound in pregnancy:

- A Detected anencephaly for the first time in 1971
- B Has reduced perinatal deaths not due to congenital abnormalities
- C Can be used to screen for Down syndrome
- D Is a safe procedure
- E Can be done in early pregnancy by use of a vaginal probe

5.55 Puerperal psychosis:

A Usually begins after the second week of the puerperium

B Often takes the form of schizophrenia

C Recurs in subsequent pregnancies as a rule

D Usually develops insidiously

E Usually has a good prognosis

5.56 Fetal size and growth:

A Is accurately measured by abdominal palpation

B Is best assessed by an ultrasound scan

C Is closely related to maternal weight gain

D Is usefully screened using fundal height measurement

E Will vary between different racial groups

5.57 With regard to *Why Mothers Die 2000–2002*, in comparison with the report from 1997–99, the overall findings for 2000–2002 shows:

A Increased deaths from thrombosis and thromboembolism

B Significant increase in deaths from haemorrhage

C Number of direct deaths is greater than the number of indirect maternal deaths

D Deaths from suicide is the leading cause of maternal deaths

E The total number of direct deaths is remarkably similar to that reported in 1997–99

5.58 Preterm rupture of membranes (PROM):

- A Occurs in 1 of 10 pregnancies after 37 weeks
- B Preterm premature rupture of the membranes (PPROM) occurs before 37 weeks and after the onset of labour
- C Can lead to premature delivery
- D Presents with the main complaint being of pelvic pressure
- E Can be managed expectantly

5.59 With regard to analgesia in labour:

- A Epidural analgesia is the most effective method
- B It is likely that epidural analgesia lengthens labour and results in increased rates of operative vaginal delivery
- C Nitrous oxide is commonly the inhalation analgesia used
- D Transcutaneous nerve stimulation (TENS) can be used in labour
- E Pethidine is a central nervous system depressant

5.60 With regard to lactation and infant feeding:

- A Breast feeding protects again gastrointestinal infection in the infant
- B Combined oestrogen-progestogen oral contraceptives should not be avoided in breast-feeding mothers
- C Oestrogen can be used to suppress lactation
- D Cabergoline is more effective than bromocriptine for the suppression of lactation and may be used as a single dose
- E Antibiotics and/or cabbage leaves are very effective for breast engorgement

EXTENDED MATCHING QUESTIONS

30 Questions: Time allowed 1 hour.

THEME: MINOR DISORDERS OF PREGNANCY

A Adrenergic agents
B Antacids
C Antihistamines
D Aspirin
E Explanation and reassurance
F Increased dietary fibre
G Lubricant laxatives
H Paracetamol
I Proton-pump inhibitors
J Support stockings

Instructions: From the list above choose the most appropriate management for each minor disorder of pregnancy given below. Each option can be used once, more than once or not at all.

5.61 A woman with severe headaches in the last trimester.

5.62 A woman with normal serum bile acids and itchy skin.

5.63 A woman with postural hypotension.

Answers on pages 335–338

THEME: HYPERTENSIVE DISEASE IN PREGNANCY

A Ask the patient to return the next day for review
B Call for an ambulance
C Prescribe antihypertensive medication and see in a week
D Refer to hospital on the same day
E Refer to hospital that week
F Refer to hospital the next day
G Review in a week's time

Instructions: A 32 weeks' pregnant primipara attends your antenatal clinic at your general practice. Her blood pressure has been normal previously. She is asymptomatic. From the list above choose the most appropriate advice for the possible situations described below. Each option can be used once, more than once or not at all.

5.64 Blood pressure is 140/90 mmHg, no proteinuria and the fetal size is clinically normal.

5.65 Blood pressure is 170/115 mmHg, 4+ proteinuria and the height of the uterine fundus approximating to a 28-week gestation.

5.66 Blood pressure is 140/100 mmHg, 1+ proteinuria and the fetal size is smaller than expected.

THEME: GESTATIONAL DIABETES

A Fasting blood glucose estimation
B Glucose tolerance test at 20–28 weeks' gestation
C Glucose tolerance test in the same week
D Refer to pregnancy/diabetes service for consultant care
E Repeat urine testing for glucose in 1 week
F Routine antenatal care

Instructions: From the list above choose the appropriate steps to take in the circumstances given below. Each option can be used once, more than once or not at all.

5.67 A 28-year-old woman with 2+ glycosuria at 16 weeks' gestation.

5.68 A 32-year-old woman at 16 weeks' gestation who was treated with insulin for gestational diabetes in her last pregnancy.

5.69 A 30-week pregnant woman whose mother has type 2 diabetes and has a 2+ glycosuria specimen for the first time in that pregnancy.

THEME: POSTPARTUM HAEMORRHAGE

A Evacuation of the uterus
B Intravenous antibiotics
C Intravenous oxytocin
D Intravenous oxytocin and antibiotics
E Hysterectomy
F No treatment
G Oral antibiotics
H Pelvic ultrasound

Instructions: From the list above choose the most appropriate management for the clinical scenarios described below. Each option can be used once, more than once or not at all.

5.70 A healthy woman, 1-week post normal delivery with ongoing daily vaginal blood loss.

5.71 A woman admitted with an acute vaginal bleed of 500 ml, 1 month after delivery.

5.72 A woman with ongoing daily bleeding for 3 weeks after caesarean delivery as well as offensive lochia and a normal temperature.

THEME: INDUCTION OF LABOUR

A Artificial rupture of membranes
B Artificial rupture of membranes + intravenous oxytocin infusion
C Do not induce labour
D Intravenous oxytocin infusion
E Membrane sweep
F Oral administration of prostaglandins
G Vaginal administration of prostaglandins

Instructions: From the list above choose the most appropriate advice that you would give to a primiparous woman with a cephalic presentation who requests an induction of labour. Each option can be used once, more than once or not at all.

5.73 A healthy woman with a healthy baby who is 40 weeks + 10 days gestation. The Bishop score is 3.

5.74 A healthy woman who has a healthy fetus with suspected macrosomia at 38 weeks' gestation.

5.75 A woman who is admitted for induction of labour with a cervix at 4 cm dilated and the membranes intact.

THEME: MENSTRUAL DISTURBANCE

A Asherman syndrome
B Conn syndrome
C Cushing syndrome
D Hypertension
E Parathyroid disease
F Thyroid disease
G Tuberculosis

Instructions: From the list above choose the most likely cause for the situations described below. Each option can be used once, more than once or not at all.

5.76 A 46-year-old woman presents with a goitre and secondary amenorrhoea.

5.77 A 36-year-old woman presents with secondary amenorrhoea after having an evacuation of the uterus for retained products of conception, 6 months ago.

5.78 A woman who has just arrived in the UK complains of weight loss, a chronic cough for 8 months and secondary amenorrhoea.

THEME: VIRAL INFECTIONS

A Herpes simplex virus (HSV) 1
B HSV 2
C Human immunodeficiency virus (HIV) 1
D HIV 2
E Human papilloma virus (HPV) 6, 8
F HPV 15, 17
G HPV 16, 18

Instructions: From the list above choose the most likely causative virus for the clinical conditions given below. Each option can be used once, more than once or not at all.

5.79 Warty lesions on vulva and perineum

5.80 Cervical cancer

5.81 Repeated painful ulcerative lesions on the labia

THEME: MENSTRUAL DISTURBANCE

A Bilateral salpingo-oophorectomy
B Combined oral contraceptive
C Endometrial ablation
D Hysterectomy
E Mirena (levonorgestrel) intrauterine system (IUS)
F Myomectomy
G Synthetic progestogens
H Tranexamic acid

Instructions: From the list above choose the most appropriate treatment for the scenarios described below. Each option can be used once, more than once or not at all.

5.82 A 46-year-old woman with menorrhagia for 8 months and a normal endometrial sample.

5.83 A 42-year-old woman with menorrhagia who has completed her family, and an ultrasound scan reveals a multiple fibroid uterus.

5.84 A 36-year-old woman with regular heavy periods who is trying to conceive.

THEME: GENERAL GYNAECOLOGY

A Bromocriptine
B Clomifene
C Gentamicin
D Hyosine
E Metformin
F Metronidazole
G Morphine
H Testosterone implant

Instructions: From the list above choose the drug treatment that matches with the clinical conditions given below. Each option can be used once, more than once or not at all.

5.85 Hyperprolactinaemia

5.86 Polycystic ovary syndrome

5.87 Bacterial vaginosis

THEME: INFERTILITY

A Adoption
B Artificial insemination by donor
C Artificial insemination by husband
D Controlled ovarian stimulation
E Intrauterine insemination
F Intracytoplasmic sperm injection
G In vitro fertilisation
H Ovum donation
I Surrogacy

Instructions: From the list above choose the most appropriate intervention to match the conditions given below. Each option can be used once, more than once or not at all.

5.88 Bilateral salpingectomy

5.89 Spinal cord injury to husband

5.90 Azoospermia

Practice Paper 5 Answers

5.1 A: Insulin

Insulin has no metabolic interactions with oral contraceptives.

5.2 E: Maternal diabetes

Maternal diabetes is not associated with postmaturity.

5.3 E: Pregnacny does not accelerate the course of HIV

HIV in pregnancy has implications for the mother and baby. Vaginal delivery is not an absolute contraindication and can be done in women with low viral load. Breast feeding, traumatic delivery and fetal blood sampling increase chances of fetal infection and therefore are contraindicated.

5.4 B: Maternal toxoplasmosis

Toxoplasma infection is not related with macrosomia, but it could be a cause of intrauterine growth restriction. All the others are associated with macrosomia.

5.5 A: Reduction in labour duration by 60–120 mins

Artificial rupture of membranes (ARM) reduces the duration of labour but may slightly increase the need for lower segment caesarean section and poor Apgar score at 5 minutes. There is no increased risk of admission to neonatal unit following ARM.

Questions on pages 279–287

5.6 E: Face presentation – mento-anterior position

Presenting diameters in mento-anterior presentations are not high, however, mento-posterior face presentation and brow can contribute to cephalopelvic disproportion. Also other abnormal presentations – shoulder, compound presentation – can contribute to cephalopelvic disproportion.

5.7 D: Routine endotracheal suctioning to clear the trachea of meconium

If the baby is active and vigorous there is no need for routine endotracheal suction as it can cause injury to the pharynx without improving outcome.

5.8 C: Episiotomy is recommended for instrumental delivery based on evidence

Episiotomy reduces the chance of anterior vaginal wall trauma and is performed to avoid perineal trauma associated with forceps, but not routinely advised in cases of ventouse delivery. There are no studies to support routine episiotomy, judgement is based on clinical need in an individual case. Forceps delivery increases risk of perineal trauma and 60% of women have sphincter defect on ultrasound.

5.9 C: Rectal temperature < 36 °C

Most infants pass urine within 24 hours. If the infant appears well investigations are not started so early. Cephalhematoma and erythema toxicum are self-limiting. Rectal temperature < 36 °C in babies should be treated as hypothermia. Breast-fed babies tend to lose slightly more weight than bottle fed infants in the first week of life.

5.10 D: Marked increase in mortality from circulatory disease

PCOS is associated with increased risk of all the conditions listed in the question, however it does not have a remarkable influence on mortality associated with circulatory disease. It is associated with increased risk of endometrial cancer and ovarian cancer.

5.11 C: Affects fallopian tube motility and therefore impairs sperm migration and ovum transport

Progesterone-only contraceptives do not have effect on fallopian tubes, although oral contraceptive may possibly have direct effect on fallopian tubes.

5.12 A: Menorrhagia and anaemia

Menorrhagia and anaemia are relative contraindications for the use of the IUCD, but the IUS (Mirena or levonorgestrel coil) is indicated in such patients. All the others are absolute contraindications.

5.13 A: 46,XXY

Men with Klinefelter syndrome are usually tall and oligozoospermic and present with subfertility.

5.14 C: Deepening of voice

Voice changes due to danazol are irreversible. Other changes due to androgenic activity of danazol usually improve once medication is stopped.

5.15 E: Duchenne muscular dystrophy

Duchenne muscular dystrophy is an X-linked disorder. All the others are autosomal recessive disorders. Other X-linked disorders are haemophilia and Lesch–Nyhan syndrome.

5.16 E: Abnormalities are detected better when performed after 20 weeks

Abnormalities are better detected at later gestation. Detection rates for neural tube defects are high. Calyceal dilatation is usually detected after 30 weeks. Rate of detection of cardiac abnormalities is about 50–60%.

5.17 B: Tramsmission of pain in first stage of labour is related to T10–T12 and L1 level

Both epidural and spinal anaesthesia can reduce the blood pressure (BP), although the epidural results in a slower fall compared with the epidural. Transmission is through the S2–S5 nerve roots in the second stage of labour. Epidural does not affect duration of labour remarkably in the first stage, however it does prolong the second stage.

5.18 E: Referral to a gynaecologist oncologist

The patient is most likely to have an ovarian malignancy (epithelial carcinoma constitutes 80% of all). She will need a laparotomy and reduction surgery (total abdominal hysterectomy + bilateral salpingo-oophorectomy + omentectomy). Suspected malignancy is best managed by a gynaecological oncologist. Serous adenocarcinoma comprises 40% of all malignant ovarian tumours. Endometrial cancers co-exist with endometrioid tumours in 20–30% of cases, therefore hysterectomy is also done. One in three serous adenocarcinomas is bilateral.

5.19 B: Ginger can be used for treatment

Hyperemesis gravidarum is associated with more successful pregnancies and with hyperthyroidism. The incidence is lower in smokers and ginger is an effective treatment.

5.20 B: Accurate diagnosis should be made by history and speculum examination

Accurate diagnosis is made based on history and speculum examination. Digital vaginal examination should be avoided unless advanced labour is suspected. Co-amoxiclav markedly increases the incidence of neonatal necrotising enterocolitis. Erythromycin improves neonatal morbidity and mortality. Induction is not considered before 37 weeks unless there is any obstetric or fetal indication to do so.

5.21 C

There is no evidence that maternal growth hormone positively influences birth weight. Primiparity and social class are not consistently related to birth weight.

5.22 ABCDE

Lie is defined as the relationship of the fetus to the long axis of mother. Cephalic presentation is the commonest presentation at term (95%).This is because of the shape of the uterine cavity which allows more room for lower limb activities in the fundal region. Any condition that alters the shape and the position of the uterus will increase the incidence of malpresentations of the fetus and increase the likelihood of unstable lie. These include multigravid uterus, polyhydramnios, prematurity, placenta praevia, fibroid, ovarian tumour in pouch of Douglas, uterine abnormalities (bicornate uterus) and fetal abnormalities such as hydrocephalus.

5.23 BDE

A hysterosalpingogram demonstrates tubal patency, which is subtly different from tubal function. It has a role in detecting uterine adhesions (Asherman syndrome). It is important in the management of infertility to make sure that the investigation itself does not cause problems. A high vaginal swab as well as an endocervical swab looking for *Chlamydia* is ideal management. Prophylactic antibiotics should also be considered. Fibroids can impinge on the cavity, increasing the risk of failure to implant, and the hysteroscope is taking over the role of the hysterosalpingogram.

Questions on pages 289–303

5.24 AD

Bilateral salpingo-oophorectomy in premenopausal women is associated with a surgical menopause, therefore, unless it is contraindicated, hormone replacement therapy is essential. This need not be given with progestogens as there is no endometrium and unopposed oestrogens could be given orally, by implant or by patch. Premenstrual syndrome is associated with ovulation and perhaps should be called ovarian cycle syndrome. It is, therefore, eliminated by bilateral salpingo-oophorectomy at the time of a hysterectomy. Oophorectomy is not usually technically more difficult than a hysterectomy unless, of course, the ovaries are buried in adhesions. In women between the age of 45 and 50 years it is usually advised to have the ovaries removed to decrease the risk not only of benign ovarian cysts and ovarian carcinoma but also of deep dyspareunia.

5.25 B

Uncomplicated vulvovaginal candidiasis affects about 75% of women at least once in their lifetime and is self-limiting. Recurrent thrush occurs in about 5% of healthy women of reproductive age. *Candida albicans* has been reported to cause 75–80% of vulvovaginal candidiasis, however, there has been an increase in the number of cases caused by *Candida glabrata* and *Candida tropicalis*. Well-known aetiological factors include:

- antibiotics
- sexual intercourse
- diabetes mellitus
- immunosuppression
- pregnancy
- combined oral contraceptive pill with high dose of oestrogen
- hormone replacement therapy
- intrauterine contraceptive devices.

Bubble bath, wearing non-cotton underwear and vaginal douching are largely anecdotal causes of vulvovaginal candidiasis and their causative role remains unproved. Vaginal pH is usually normal (pH 3.5–4.5). If the pH is raised, a diagnosis of trichomoniasis or bacterial vaginosis should be considered.

5.26 BCDE

Dysmenorrhoea (ie painful menstruation) may be primary or secondary and is a distinctly different problem from premenstrual syndrome. Primary dysmenorrhoea occurs in young women with the onset of the ovulation cycle and without any specific underlying pathology. Abnormal levels of prostaglandins cause excessive uterine contractions. The pill is a useful form of treatment. Secondary dysmenorrhoea occurs in older women and results from underlying pelvic pathology, such as endometriosis, intrauterine contraceptive device, chronic pelvic inflammatory disease, or fibroids.

5.27 ABCE

Monozygotic twins occur at a rate of about 1:260 and this rate is constant with no known predisposing factors. The incidence of dizygotic twins is influenced by:

- Race – Nigerians have a risk of about 1:20 per birth, whereas the risk in Europeans is about 1:80.
- Inheritance – a family history of twins on the mother's side is still closely associated with increased risk of twinning.
- Both increasing maternal age and parity are associated with a twin pregnancy.
- Induction of ovulation – not only does clomifene and the use of gonadotrophins increase the risk of twins, but in vitro fertilisation is also associated with an increased risk of twins. The Human Fertilisation and Embryology Authority recommends that two embryos should be transferred, three in exceptional circumstances and this has reduced the twinning rates.

... continued

There are many complications of twinning and they are basically associated with increased risk of all the medical problems in pregnancy. Because of the increase in placental size there is also a risk of placenta praevia.

5.28 ACD

In vitro fertilisation and ovum donation do not require patent tubes because the embryo is transferred back directly into the uterine cavity. The other methods require patent tubes in order to allow fertilisation to take place.

5.29 ACD

All types of intrauterine contraceptive device lead to an increase in the number of leukocytes, not only in the endometrium but also in the uterine and tubal fluids. Inert and copper devices lead to an increase in the levels of many prostaglandins. Copper enhances this foreign body reaction and leads to a range of biochemical changes in the endometrium affecting the enzyme system and hormone receptors. These copper ions are toxic to the sperm and blastocyst. Progestogen-releasing coils are now becoming more popular and are also useful in heavy periods. Inert devices are no longer available in the UK. As the surface area of the inert device is reduced so the side-effects of bleeding and pain are minimised but the failure rate increases. With the introduction of copper, a smaller device can be used without this loss of efficiency. The levonorgestrel device reduces menstrual blood flow, but the copper-containing devices do not. The intrauterine contraceptive device is a highly effective method which:

- is nearly always reversible
- does not have any known systemic side-effects
- is independent of intercourse
- does not require much motivation or day-to-day action
- is relatively cheap
- is easy to distribute
- does not affect the postpartum mother.

5.30 CE

From mid-pregnancy onwards the fetal kidney contributes increasingly to amniotic fluid volume, contributing some 500 ml/day by term; in renal agenesis the liquor volume is greatly reduced. The volume of amniotic fluid may be estimated by ultrasound but not accurately. Liquor volumes are higher than average in rhesus-affected pregnancies and grossly increased in hydrops fetalis. Amniocentesis may permit amniotic fluid to leak away, thus reducing the volume. Pre-eclampsia and intrauterine growth retardation are both associated with reduced amniotic fluid volumes.

5.31 ABD

Heartburn is a common condition in pregnancy. It is important to be aware that in late pregnancy it can be associated with pre-eclampsia and the HELLP (Haemolysis, Elevated Liver enzymes and Low Platelets) syndrome. It has the same pathophysiology as pre-eclampsia but may not have the initial rise in blood pressure. A useful screen blood test includes: liver function test, full blood count to include platelets, urea and electrolytes, urate.

5.32 DE

Biophysical profiling which measures fetal movement, tone, reactivity of the heart, breathing and amniotic fluid volume may be a better predictor of fetal compromise than cardiotocography alone. At present, it is a time consuming and costly test and may not be appropriate as a screening test for fetal compromise. Although fetal biophysical profiling is a better predictor of low 5-minute Apgar scores than the non-stress test cardiotocogram, it does not, in its own right, reduce the perinatal mortality rate. Doppler blood flow assessment is now becoming routine clinical practice.

5.33 ACE

Condylomata acuminata, otherwise known as genital warts, are due to papillomavirus. Bartholinitis is usually caused by coliform organisms or staphylococci. Cervical intraepithelial neoplasia (CIN) is thought to be caused by human papillomavirus, type 16. Lichen sclerosus is a type of vulval dystrophy of unknown aetiology. Acute vulval ulcers are most commonly due to infection with the herpes virus.

5.34 ABE

The most common symptom of cervical cancer is abnormal vaginal bleeding (such as postcoital bleeding, intermenstrual bleeding and postmenopausal bleeding). Studies have shown that human papillomavirus infection is the major risk factor for development of preinvasive or invasive carcinoma of the cervix, which far outweighs other known risk factors such as increasing number of sexual partners, young age at first intercourse, low socioeconomic status, and positive smoking history. There were 2740 new cases of invasive cervical cancer in England and Wales in 1997 (9.3 cases per 100 000 women). The UK has the second highest recorded incidence in the European Union. Deaths from cervical cancer have fallen by more than 40% from 7.0 deaths per 100 000 in 1979 to 4.1 per 100 000 in 1995. Cervical cancer is the twelfth most common cause of cancer deaths in women in the UK.

5.35 BCE

Pregnancy induces a haemodilution effect on the blood and, therefore, the normal haemoglobin adaptations that occur with pregnancy may be inappropriately diagnosed as iron deficiency. Mean cell volume may be the most useful parameter for assessing iron deficiency as it falls quite rapidly in the presence of decreased iron. There is no good evidence that the addition of molybdenum, ascorbic acid, copper, or manganese improves the efficacy of iron. A megaloblastic anaemia in pregnancy is nearly always associated with folate deficiency with evidence of late-stage folate deficiency. Under these circumstances rapid blood changes occur with folic acid supplementation.

5.36 ACE

The oral contraceptive has few side-effects. By increasing sex-hormone-binding-globulins it increases the bound testosterone and, therefore, decreases the testosterone activity. Danazol has an androgenic effect. Cyproterone acetate is most effective working at the level of the hair follicles as an anti-androgen and also decreasing gonadotrophin production. It needs to be given in an adequate dose and in a reversed sequential regimen. There is no evidence that electrolysis increases the risk of further hair growth.

5.37 BC

Adequate contraception is important during the climacteric – the transitional phase during which ovarian function gradually ceases around the time of the final menstrual period (the menopause). Levels of follicle-stimulating hormone (FSH) greater than 30 IU/l are usually suggestive of ovarian failure but one also has to be cautious about the diagnosis of resistant ovaries which can spontaneously ovulate. Reliable measurement of FSH can be difficult when a woman is taking a combined oral contraceptive or taking hormone replacement therapy (HRT). HRT cannot be relied on as a contraceptive because ovulation may still occur.

5.38 A

Vulval carcinoma is associated with pruritus vulvae. Pruritus vulvae is, however, a common problem associated with lichen sclerosus. Carcinoma of the vulva is increasing, but this is possibly associated with increasing life expectancy. Carcinoma of the vulva is usually unifocal, although it can be multifocal when 'KISS' lesions are noted. It is much more common in African patients and there is no association with parity. The treatment of choice is surgical.

5.39 ACDE

Abruption is a known complication of polyhydramnios due to the sudden decompression of the uterus at rupture of the membranes. It is essential when performing amniotomy to ensure that there is a slow release of the amniotic fluid. Intrauterine growth retardation results from poor uterine blood flow which causes placental insufficiency and oligohydramnios. Oesophageal atresia prevents effective fetal swallowing and therefore excessive amniotic fluid forms. The over-distended uterus is more irritable and prone to preterm labour. The overstretched uterus does not retract and therefore post-partum haemorrhage is a complication in cases of polyhydramnios.

5.40 ABD

A progestogen is a steroid which causes a withdrawal bleed on an oestrogen-primed endometrium. If, when given to a postmenopausal woman, it induces a withdrawal bleed, endometrial hyperplasia should be suspected. Traditional treatment with cyclical oral progestogen is of limited efficiency in menorrhagia during ovulatory cycles, unless the cycles are short. In this case, progestogens can help to delay the onset of bleeding. In prolonged cycles, progestogens may be useful, but side-effects are common, and these include weight gain, nausea, bloating and headaches. Norethisterone has androgenic properties; medroxyprogesterone acetate and dydrogesterone are non-androgenic alternatives. Postmenopausal women are at risk of endometrial hyperplasia. If no uterus is present then unopposed oestrogen treatment is appropriate.

5.41 ABD

Elective lower segment caesarean section is performed at 39 weeks. The highest morbidity and mortality is associated with footling breech presentation.

5.42 ABD

Pyelonephritis should be treated with antibiotics for at least 14 days. Amoxicillin or cephalosporins are first line of drug for treatment in pregnancy.

5.43 AC

Less than 5% become symptomatic. Visual field testing is needed only for patients with symptoms of headache or visual disturbance. Breast feeding is not contraindicated. Prolactin levels are normally raised in pregnancy therefore unhelpful in diagnosis.

5.44 ABC

Universal screening is offered to all pregnant women in the UK. The rate of transmission is reduced to < 2% with appropriate interventions.

5.45 BCD

Rubella vaccination is avoided in pregnant women until the postnatal period if the woman is found to be antibody negative. Cholera vaccine is not a prerequisite as it does not prevent the spread of disease.

5.46 ABE

Limb reduction can occur following early chorionic villus sampling.

5.47 ABC

Carboprost is an oxytocic and causes strong uterine contractions and is used for the management of postpartum haemorrhage. Ergometrine is also used after delivery.

5.48 BCD

Uterine hyperstimulation not hypostimulation can result from induction. Neonatal jaundice and water intoxication can occur due to excessive use of oxytocin. Fetal distress could arise from the overuse of oxytocin without adequate monitoring of contractions.

5.49 BC

Normal baseline is 110–160 beats/min. There should be two accelerations in a 20-minute period. The cardiotocograph has a poor long-term prognostic value.

5.50 AE

A vaginal examination in active labour for a low-risk patient is performed every 4 hours. Active management of third stage is by giving Syntometrine at delivery of shoulder.

5.51 ADE

There are three inter-related indications for the use of low-dose aspirin in pregnancy:

- For pre-eclampsia prophylaxis – this is limited at present to those who are judged to be at risk of early onset of pre-eclampsia.
- Management of primary antiphospholipid syndrome which is associated with an increased risk of first- and second-trimester fetal loss, and also when at risk of thromboembolism, not only venous but also arterial.
- Thromboprophylaxis, although at present no randomised control study has been performed to confirm this.

5.52 ABCD

Gardnerella vaginalis is a Gram-negative bacillus. It is associated with bacterial vaginosis. Diagnosis can be difficult but is aided by the following:

- There is a disagreeable, fishy smell, particularly after intercourse
- Clue cells, which are bacteria attached to the vaginal epithelial cells, are present
- the vaginal pH is > 5: this is associated with both *Gardnerella* and *Trichomonas.*
- *Gardnerella* can be transported on Stuart's medium.

5.53 ABCD

Women who develop thrush following antibiotic treatment should be given anti-thrush agents prophylactically. Aqueous creams can be used as a soap substitute as well as an emollient for the vulval skin. Several studies have shown the effectiveness of maintenance treatment with antifungals once an induction regimen has effected a cure. Maintenance treatment for up to six months includes:

- Fluconazole – 100 mg weekly
- Itraconazole – 50–100 mg/day
- Ketoconazole –100 mg/day
- Clotrimazole – per vaginam weekly

Resistant yeasts can be treated with vaginal boric acid 600 mg daily for 14 days or topical flucytosine. Injections of medroxyprogesterone acetate have been used.

5.54 ACDE

Routine ultrasonography is beneficial to confirm gestational age early on and to look for congenital abnormalities between 16 and 20 weeks. The role of nuchal fold thickness scanning is being evaluated at present and has its uses as a screening test for Down syndrome. Although the ultrasound scan is helpful in the management of pregnancy, including the confirmation of dates, and the detection of twins, blighted ovum and hydatidiform mole, it is yet to reduce perinatal deaths not due to congenital abnormalities.

5.55 E

Puerperal psychosis usually begins within the first 7–10 days of the puerperium and most often takes the form of depression. Schizophrenia or mania are rare. The onset is often acute and the eventual outcome good. The risk of recurrence in subsequent pregnancies is between 1:3 and 1:7.

5.56 BDE

Fetal growth and size are very difficult to assess. The measurement by abdominal palpation is extremely crude and some people would even describe it as a blind guess. Clinically, the most widely practised techniques are measurement of the fundal height and of the abdominal girth at the level of the umbilicus. Several studies have shown good sensitivity and specificity of fundal height for detecting low birth weight for gestation. It is, therefore, a useful screening test which can detect growth restriction. Maternal weight gain is of limited importance. Ultrasound is generally considered to be the best available method of measuring fetal size and growth.

5.57 BDE

During this triennium there have been a decreases in deaths from thrombosis and thromboembolism. This may be because of the routine introduction and use of guidelines which were introduced as a result of the recommendations from previous CEMD Reports.

Haemorrhage deaths have increased from 7 to 17.

The number of indirect deaths (155), due to pre-existing disease aggravated by pregnancy, is greater than deaths directly related to pregnancy (106).

Suicide is the leading cause of maternal death when deaths up to 1 year after delivery are included.

The number of direct deaths was also 106 in the previous report

5.58 AE

The incidence of preterm rupture of membranes (PROM) is approximately 10% of pregnancies. The terminology can be confusing. PROM is rupture of the membranes (ROM) prior to the onset of labour in a woman who is beyond 37 weeks' gestation. Preterm premature rupture of the membranes (PPROM) is ROM prior to the onset of labour in a woman who is less than 37 weeks' gestation. Women with PROM may present with the chief complaints of leaking fluid and vaginal discharge. PPROM is associated with 30% of preterm deliveries, not PROM. Several studies have reported that expectant management decreased the rate of caesarean delivery and length of labour without increasing the rate of infection, especially in cases with an unfavourable cervix. The woman's desires should always be considered and the management options should be discussed with her, with careful documentation.

5.59 ABCDE

Epidural analgesia is the most effective method of analgesia in labour. It often slows the second stage by reducing or eliminating the normal surge of oxytocin and by reducing pelvic floor muscle tone. This may lead to more instrumental deliveries. A mixture of nitrous oxide and oxygen is one of the most common methods of obstetric analgesia that maintains consciousness. 'Entonox' is a 50:50 mixture of the two gases and acts on the central nervous system, resulting initially in analgesia and later in anaesthesia. Entonox takes 30 seconds to act and its effect continues for approximately 60 seconds after inhalation has ceased. Transcutaneous nerve stimulation (TENS) produces electrical stimulation and provides distraction while simultaneously gating the pain impulses at the level of the spinal cord. Pethidine is a central nervous system depressant. This drug has an onset of action of about 15 minutes and a duration of action of 2–4 hours. A standard dose is 50–100 mg intramuscularly, repeated 1–3 hours later if necessary.

5.60 AD

Breast feeding, compared with artificial feeding, has been clearly shown to protect against gastrointestinal infection in the infant and against necrotising enterocolitis among babies born at more than 30 weeks' gestation. Combined oestrogen-progestogen oral contraceptives should be avoided during breast feeding as they could increase the incidence of breast-feeding failure. Oestrogen should not be used for lactation suppression as it increases the risk of vaginal bleeding and of thromboembolism. For those who have lost a baby, pharmacological suppression of lactation may be considered: bromocriptine is effective in lactation suppression but rebound lactation is common. Cabergoline is more effective than bromocriptine and may be used as a single dose. In simple breast engorgement, antibiotics and oxytocin are unlikely to be beneficial. Unrestricted access for the baby to the breast still appears to be the most effective way to prevent and treat breast engorgement, prematurity and/or low birth weight.

EXTENDING MATCHING QUESTIONS ANSWERS

THEME: MINOR DISORDERS OF PREGNANCY

5.61 H Paracetamol and not aspirin may be used sparingly.

5.62 E Explanation and reassurance. There is no effective treatment for itchy skin.

5.63 E Explanation and reassurance is all that is needed as there are no adverse obstetric consequences of this problem.

THEME: HYPERTENSIVE DISEASE IN PREGNANCY

5.64 A Ask the patient to return the next day for review. The chance find of raised blood pressure and no proteinuria needs to be confirmed before referral.

5.65 B Call for an ambulance. This is a potentially severe situation and prompt, supervised referral to hospital is warranted. There is a risk of eclampsia and need for emergency management in hospital.

5.66 D Refer to hospital on the same day. Same day referral is needed as the fetal condition needs to be assessed before a management plan is devised.

Questions on pages 305–314

THEME: GESTATIONAL DIABETES

5.67 C Glucose tolerance test the same week. A single episode of glycosuria before 20 weeks' gestation should be followed up by an estimation of blood glucose, either a timed/random sample or a glucose tolerance test. (National Institute for Health and Clinical Excellence guidelines do not advocate testing for glycosuria.)

5.68 B Glucose tolerance test at 20–28 weeks' gestation. Previous gestational diabetes is a risk factor for the re-occurrence in a future pregnancy.

5.69 C Glucose tolerance test the same week. There are two risk factors, a first-degree family relative and glycosuria, and they are indications for a glucose tolerance test. The glucose tolerance test needs to be performed quickly so an appropriate management plan can be instituted.

THEME: POSTPARTUM HAEMORRHAGE

5.70 F No treatment. This is normal lochia and should progressively decrease.

5.71 D Intravenous oxytocin and antibiotics should be the initial treatment. Further investigation and possibly evacuation may be undertaken after the initial treatment.

5.72 G Oral antibiotics. Retained products of conception are unlikely after a caesarean section. The diagnosis is endometritis and antibiotics are needed.

THEME: INDUCTION OF LABOUR

5.73 G Induction of labour after 41 weeks reduces the perinatal mortality rate and does not increase the caesarean section rate. Compared with oxytocin regimens, the induction of labour with prostaglandins results in a reduction in epidural and caesarean section rates and an increase in the chance of successful delivery in 24 hours.

5.74 C There is no proved benefit of inducing labour for suspected macrosomia in women who are not diabetic.

5.75 B Rupture of membranes should precede an oxytocin infusion to increase the efficiency of the induction.

THEME: MENSTRUAL DISTURBANCE

5.76 F Thyroid disease.

5.77 A This is a classic presentation of Asherman syndrome.

5.78 G Chronic illnesses such as tuberculosis can cause amenorrhoea and recent immigrants to the UK fall into the high-risk groups and need to undergo investigations whenever they present with such symptoms.

THEME: VIRAL INFECTIONS

5.79 E HPV 6 and 8 cause viral warts.

5.80 G HPV 16 and 18 are oncogenic subtypes and cause high-grade cervical intraepithelial neoplasia (CIN) lesions and are found in 99% of cancer of the cervix cases

5.81 B HSV 2 causes herpes genitalis and HSV 1 causes herpes labialis.

THEME: MENSTRUAL DISTURBANCE

5.82 E Mirena IUS reduces menstrual blood loss by 97% at 12 months. It is contraceptive and is effective for 5 years.

5.83 D Hysterectomy is a definitive cure for menorrhagia reserved for a woman who has completed her family.

5.84 H Tranexamic acid is an inhibitor of fibrinolysis. Its effects are dose related, and it can reduce menstrual blood loss by 50%. It can be taken with heavy periods.

THEME: GENERAL GYNAECOLOGY

5.85 A Bromocriptine can shrink microadenomas and reduce prolactin levels leading to clinical improvement.

5.86 E There is emerging data that metformin controls the endocrinopathy in polycystic ovary syndrome and leads to high chances of ovulation and higher rates of fertility.

5.87 F Metronidazole.

THEME: INFERTILITY

5.88 G In vitro fertilisation.

5.89 C Artificial insemination by husband.

5.90 F Intracytoplasmic sperm injection.

Index

Locators refer to the question number.